Twelve & Se7vn

By
Brenda J Farah Coleman

Table of Contents

About the Author

Brenda J. Farah Coleman

Brenda J. Farah Coleman is an American writer and the author of *TWELVE & SE7VEN*, a powerful and deeply personal reflection on faith, healing, and the resilience of the human spirit. Her writing is shaped by a lifetime of extraordinary experiences—both professional and personal—that have allowed her to understand people with uncommon depth and empathy.

Before becoming an author, Brenda built an accomplished career serving the United States through her work in the Department of Defense. As a Human Resource Subject Matter Expert (SME) and Officer HR PRO, she managed officer records, contributed to HR Basic Trainee enlistment operations, and helped maintain the standards and systems that support America's military personnel. Her commitment to service and her dedication to excellence defined her years within the Department of Defense, leaving a lasting impact on military personnel and their families.

Brenda has also excelled as a communications professional and is a licensed cosmetologist—careers that reflect her natural ability to connect with people from all walks of life. Whether she is mentoring, advising, comforting, or uplifting others, Brenda carries a unique gift for understanding human behavior and offering compassion where it is needed most.

Among all her achievements, one role stands above the rest: being an aunt. Brenda proudly embraces her position as "Auntie" not only to her biological nieces and nephews but to many children and young adults who see her as family. Her love, protection, and guidance have shaped countless lives, and she regards this bond as one of her most meaningful accomplishments.

TWELVE & SE7VEN is more than a book—it is a testament to Brenda's journey of survival, faith, and divine purpose. Through her writing, she invites readers to walk alongside her through the challenges, revelations, and miracles that defined her path. Her story stands as a reminder that God's grace is present in every chapter of life, especially the ones that hurt the most.

Brenda J. Farah Coleman continues to inspire others through her testimony, her courage, and her unwavering belief that every trial carries a purpose and every life carries a calling.

Volume 1
The Heart of Madea's Home

This memoir recalls early childhood memories centered around Madea, the family matriarch whose home was a hub of warmth, tradition, and togetherness in Clarksdale, Mississippi. The narrative describes the daily routines, holiday celebrations, and the nurturing environment Madea created—marked by home-cooked meals, colorful aprons stitched by her hand (no machine), and her gentle guidance. The author reflects on the loss of Madea and Grandaddy, the impact of their absence, and how their stories and love laid the foundation of family strength and belonging.

The loss of Madea—and Grandaddy before her—left a profound absence in our lives. Their stories, kindness, and unwavering love became the bedrock of our family's strength. Even as grief settled over us, the foundation they built remained, offering comfort and a sense of belonging that carried us through sorrow and into gratitude for the memories they left behind.

Madea's days began early. Her hands were always busy—kneading dough, folding laundry. Her voice, gentle yet unwavering, could hush any quarrel or coax a smile from the sullenest face. Family was everything in Madea's world. Her house was the center of gravity—a sanctuary where she and Granddaddy resided with four grandchildren whom they raised, along with daily visits from their children and grandchildren. I heard aunts and cousins arriving unannounced, bringing stories, laughter, and sometimes tears.

Under Madea's watchful eye, everyone experienced a sense of inclusion—not only within the family but also as part of a tradition observed during times of both difficulty and celebration. Her stories stitched together the fragments of our past, giving shape to memories that would outlast her presence. It was in those days, surrounded by kinfolk and the warmth of Madea's kitchen, that the foundations of our family's strength were quietly laid. Everyone gathered around her, drawn by her warm spirit. Madea was gentle and soft-spoken, yet her presence commanded respect as the family matriarch. The scent of cakes and pies filled the air as they sat on her back porch.

Madea affectionately called me her "baby chick," noting how my timid nature reminded her of the little chickens that roamed in her backyard. She was always attentive to my feelings, recognizing my fear of the boys and the discomfort I found in Bea's words. Whenever Madea wanted to know if I was in my favorite spot, she would ask Shirley Jean, and the answer echoed from all the family members—an enthusiastic "yes," affirming both their attention and my cherished place within the household.

Madea was aware when the boys teased me, and she could see that it made me sad. In those moments, she would quietly place a piece of cheese, carefully shaped, into my hand and gently guide it to my mouth. I would hold onto that cheese as if it were the most precious thing I owned. I remember that the cheese always came from blocks neatly packaged in boxes—a small but meaningful detail in those comforting memories.

People from the surrounding area often visited Madea's home, knowing that everyone would receive a meal, along with a slice of pie or cake. Upon reflection, it is evident that Madea was committed to preserving Grandaddy's legacy for me. She regularly described how Grandaddy assumed responsibility for my care when I was just six weeks old, enabling the rest of the family to participate in the Christmas celebrations. Madea also noted that Shirley Jean brought me to her and Grandaddy's residence as she prepared to join the family gathering. Bea directed Shirley Jean to put me to sleep and lay me next to Grandaddy, who preferred not to attend the festival. Since no babysitter was available, this arrangement allowed everyone else to participate. Madea and Bea recognized the close relationship between Shirley Jean and Grandaddy, knowing he would always accommodate her requests regardless of the situation. Grandaddy went to heaven when I was one year old. Madea wanted me to remember him.

Thanksgiving arrives, and the entire family feels the weight of Madea's absence. Despite the sorrow, everyone finds ways to comfort one another, drawing on the traditions that Madea established for Thanksgiving. Her spirit lingers in gestures of kindness—an extra helping passed around the table, a gentle word, or a shared smile—rooted in the rituals she nurtured. This year, however, is marked not only by grief but also by gratitude for the cherished memories she left behind.

As the seasons turned without the warmth of Madea's presence, the house felt different—quieter, as if the walls themselves missed the sound of her laughter. We moved through the routines she had once orchestrated, but the rhythm felt uncertain, and sometimes even the sunlight through the curtains seemed subdued. Family gatherings continued, yet an unspoken ache hovered in the air, a longing for the gentle authority and kindness that once anchored us all.

In the hush after a story, in the sharing of a meal, I found a quiet strength and a growing understanding that Madea's presence endured—not as a shadow, but as a light carried on by those she loved.

Madea: Jane Mcgee Curtis

Grandaddy: Dave Curtis

Clarksdale, Mississippi.

They had eight children:

3 Boys:

Edgar Curtis

Dave Curtis Jr.

Alexander Curtis

Five Girls:

- Ruth Lee Curtis-Walker— (Aunt Rub)
- Addie Beatrice Curtis-Coleman (my mother Bea) — Husband: Elbert Mack Coleman
- Beaulah Curtis-Collins (Aunt Kochie) — Husband: Cleo Collins
- Dorthy Curtis-Burnetta (Aunt Foots)
- Barbara Jean Cunningham (Aunt Bobby Jean) — Husband: CW Cunningham
- Raised 4 Grandchildren: Janie Curtis, Roy Curtis, William Curtis (Red), Lerlene Curtis (2girls, 2 boys)
-
-

My Mother: Addie Beatrice Curtis Coleman (Bea)

Bea had five children by Five different fathers.

Charles William Curtis, who changed his last name to match that of his biological father, Charles William Franklin

Katie Louise Curtis (Carter) — Husband John Carter

Lewis Curtis — lived in multiple homes, sometimes with Bea, sometimes with family on his dad's side

David Lee Curtis — resided in the family home with Bea; he and Katie were known to be Bea's favorite children

Shirley Jean Curtis — Bea's fifth born, youngest of the five, 5mos old when Bea Marriage Elbert Mack Coleman

Together, Bea and Elbert Mack Coleman had seven children:

Gloria Montgomery (Missie), First born of Bea and Elbert Coleman,

George Eddie Coleman (twin son) second

Joyce Mary Coleman (twin daughter) thirdborn

Frank Earl Coleman, fourth born

Larry Martin Coleman, fifth born

Katherine Ann Coleman (Kathy) six born

Multinominal Brenda Jean Farah Coleman Seven born Bunion, Little Chick, Farah, Little Bea, Brenda Jean, and Baby Girl — she answered to each of these names, reflecting the warmth and familiarity that surrounded her within the family.

The Heart of Grandma Mae

Grandma Mae was born on an Indian reservation in Alexandria, Louisiana, and identified as a Native American. Throughout her life, Grandma Mae and Dad often communicated using secret code words. These coded conversations reflected the inherited values central to their lives, especially as they navigated the back roads of Louisiana. Their unique way of speaking underscored the cultural traditions and resourcefulness that shaped their daily experiences.

She spent her youth working on the shore, watching boats from faraway places arrive. It was during this period, while engaged in her daily work by the shore, that she formed a relationship with a Frenchman who frequently traveled through the area and worked the shores.

As a result of that relationship, she conceived. Grandma Mae's life underwent a profound transformation upon learning she was pregnant. In accordance with her tribe's customs, this circumstance led to her being ostracized by the reservation community. Forced to leave her home while still expecting her child, she faced the daunting reality of isolation from her family and a painful separation from her roots. This period was marked by significant uncertainty, as she found herself with no one to turn to for support.

After giving birth to her son, Grandma Mae demonstrated remarkable determination and strength. She took on a variety of jobs to support herself and her child, never wavering in her commitment to provide for him. Her willingness to assume multiple roles during this challenging period displayed her resilience and dedication as a mother.

It was during these years that she met Mckinley Coleman, an older local man who would become an important part of her life. Following their marriage, Grandma Mae's son's last name was changed to Coleman, though Mckinley Coleman did not formally adopt him. Despite this, the family began their journey together, leaving their former home and venturing into the backwoods. Eventually, their travels led them to Mississippi, where they sought to build a new life as a family.

In Mississippi, they settled in the country, where Grandma Mae found the freedom to live according to the culture of her native land. This move allowed her to reconnect with her roots and embrace her heritage in ways that had previously been denied to her.

Despite these hardships, Grandma Mae remained outspoken and deeply connected to her new home in the country, far away from her native land and family. Her resilience shaped the environment she created, rooted in determination and independence.

Mary Coleman, Grandma Mae (step) Grandpa Mckinley Coleman

Mary Coleman is the mother of two children, each with a different father.

Grandma Mae's first-born son is Elbert Mack (Coleman), my father.

Grandma Mae and Grandpa had a daughter named Mary Coleman, who was Dad's sister.

Chapter 1:
The Girl Behind the Door

(Finding Comfort in Shadows)

Prior to turning four, every morning followed a familiar routine—there was never a day that did not include a visit to Bea's mom, Madea's house. The pattern was so ingrained that it felt automatic, a part of daily life that could not be separated from the start of each day.

My mother, whom everyone addressed as Bea at her request, instructed me to either wake Shirley Jean or settle into my favorite place with my doll Sam, surrounded by my coloring books and puzzles.

Bea's familiar call for my sister, Shirley Jean, signaled that she and Dad were heading off to work. This announcement marked the official beginning of our day. As soon as Bea's voice faded, Shirley Jean would call out for me, and together, we would begin our morning preparations. We would clean up and dress. After breakfast, Shirley Jean would check to make sure everyone had finished their chores.

I was confused about who lived in our house and who lived with Madea. It was the same people I saw at Madea's home. Even though mornings were always busy, Shirley Jean and I were consistently the last to arrive at Madea's. She understood that my knees often caused me discomfort, especially when I tried to walk too quickly. The friction between my bones sometimes created a burning sensation that caused redness, making it difficult for me to keep up with others.

Bea decided that my recurring knee discomfort warranted a doctor's visit. Shirley Jean and I went to see Dr. Burnham, who was the doctor present at my birth. I often visited him for shots. The doctor explained that my condition was common among children between the ages of three and six. He reassured me that my knees would straighten naturally as I grew older—by the time I reached seven or eight years old. There was no need for medical intervention; time and growth would resolve the issue.

He demonstrated how I should walk with my legs apart to reduce discomfort, emphasizing the importance of persistence and patience in adopting this new way of moving.

After our visit, Shirley Jean became even more attentive to my needs, especially as she noticed how Bea would sometimes lose her patience with me. When Bea raised her voice or called me names— which I did not understand—it often made me cry, leaving me confused and hurt. Shirley Jean devoted her time to helping me practice walking in the way the doctor recommended. With her steady support and clear instructions, I found it much easier to manage my discomfort and adapt to the new way of moving.

Despite her patience, Shirley Jean would occasionally grow tired of my slow pace. On those days, she would scoop me up and carry me the rest of the way to Madea's house, ensuring we would arrive sooner rather than later.

This morning felt different from all the others. I sat in my favorite spot, waiting for Shirley Jean to get ready as we always did, preparing to visit Madea's house. But today—we weren't going.

Dad told Shirley Jean to gather my things because I would be going to the country to visit Grandma Mae and Grandpa. He and Bea were going to Madea's house. The boys were also at home, since no one was going to Madea's as part of the usual morning routine.

I asked Shirley Jean, "Are we going to Madea's house?"

The absence of our visit hung over everyone, casting a quiet mood throughout the house. Shirley Jean told me she was going to Madea's to help take care of her because she was bed-sick.

Dad mentioned that I would be staying for a couple of days, although Grandma Mae always called it "weeks." The distinction between days and weeks always confused me, so I was never sure how long my stay would last. Despite the uncertainty, my excitement for the trip never faded.

With care, I gathered my coloring book and puzzle, holding my doll Sam close so nothing important would be forgotten. Dad made a stop at Madea's house so Bea could tend to her while he drove me out to the country.

When we arrived at Grandma Mae's home, she welcomed us warmly and led me to the bedroom so I could put away my belongings. Meanwhile, she and Dad began their conversation in another room.

Once I finished unpacking, I joined them in the front room, clutching my doll Sam tightly. Grandma Mae noticed me and gave a gentle chuckle, turning to Grandpa with a knowing smile. She commented that she already knew I would never leave Sam behind. Her laughter filled the room with warmth.

Dad offered a reassuring smile and said he would return in a couple of days. As he spoke, Grandma Mae laughed and asked me how long I would be staying—days or weeks. I shrugged my shoulders, uncertain of the answer. Grandma Mae responded with a playful remark, saying my dad didn't know either. Both grandparents shared a laugh, their warmth easing any worries I might have felt.

I don't know how long I was at Grandma Mae's. One morning, while she was making breakfast, she gently told me that Madea had gone to heaven to be with Grandaddy. I remembered she had previously said Grandaddy was in heaven, but she hadn't said Madea was going to visit him. Feeling confused, I looked to Grandma Mae for more explanation. She reassured me, saying that Shirley Jean would help me understand.

I'm not sure exactly how long I stayed, but I remember that before I returned home, Grandma Mae and Grandpa surprised me—it was my birthday. Grandma Mae prepared a vanilla cream cake with strawberries and told me I was four years old. She and Grandpa sang "Happy Birthday." Later, Dad arrived and commented that I was getting older. Grandma Mae hugged me and said I was still a baby.

Dad told me that Bea wanted me home to celebrate my birthday. Tears welled up because I did not want to leave my grandparents' house, but Grandma Mae comforted me and assured me I would return soon. Dad carried me to his truck while Grandma Mae and Grandpa packed my birthday cake and gifts, giving me hugs and kisses before we left.

When we arrived home, Dad carried me to the door and had me wait while he brought my cake and presents inside. Shirley Jean opened the door and greeted me with a bright "Happy Birthday!" She asked how old I was, and I proudly held up four fingers. She clapped her hands joyfully and told Bea she had taught me to show my age before I left for the country.

Dad showed Shirley Jean and Bea the gifts and cake I had received from my grandparents. He placed everything on the table before giving me the presents he and Bea had picked out: new clothes and a pair of shoes. Shirley Jean gifted me a comb and brush set for my doll Sam and proudly showed the cake she had baked for me.

As everyone gathered, Bea commented to Dad that his mother should have told her about baking a cake, adding that Shirley Jean didn't need to make another one. Despite her tone, the atmosphere remained cheerful. Soon my brother David Lee came home with gifts—a set of coloring books and a puzzle. Bea smiled and said, "I'm glad you didn't bring another cake." David Lee laughed and said, "Oh well, she must have all the cakes." I eagerly accepted each present, my excitement growing.

When I returned home, I sensed heaviness in the air. The usually lively atmosphere had shifted. Everyone seemed weighed down by sadness because Madea had passed—she had gone to heaven to be with Grandaddy. Although I noticed their grief, I struggled to understand it. To my mind, being together in heaven sounded joyful, not sad.

Trying to make sense of their emotions, I clung to my gifts from my grandparents. Seeking comfort, I slipped away to my favorite place. Surrounded by the things I loved most, I found solace even as I tried to understand the changes happening in my family.

Shirley Jean called for me so everyone could have a piece of cake. As we gathered around the table, Shirley Jean teased me by asking if she could have another slice. With a chuckle, she admitted Grandma Mae's cake tasted better than hers. Her laughter created a comforting atmosphere.

I heard the loud voices of the boys as they entered. Unsure of their place in our family, I asked Shirley Jean why they didn't go home. She explained gently that they lived with us and were my brothers, just like David Lee. I hadn't realized this because I was too young to understand before.

When they entered the kitchen, they asked loudly who the cakes were for. Dad and the others seemed to understand their conversations, but their intensity always made me uncomfortable. Shirley Jean told them it was my birthday, and they rushed to get plates, helping themselves to both cakes.

I slipped away to my quiet spot. Playing with Sam and using my new coloring books and puzzle brought me happiness. I fell asleep until Shirley Jean woke me for my bath and bedtime.

Later, I overheard Dad speaking to Bea about the boys. He was frustrated because they wouldn't listen when he asked them to stop wrestling. Bea grew tense, becoming protective of them anytime their behavior was mentioned. It became clear that some topics were better left unspoken. Their disagreements about discipline created strain in the house, adding to my confusion and making me keep my distance from Bea.

One time, while walking to the corner store with Bea, I saw something moving ahead of us. I tried to get her attention, but she pulled me along, saying it was only my shadow—a concept I didn't understand. On the way back, I looked for it again, and Bea said it was now behind us. I turned and saw it. She told me to focus on my knees, not the shadow. When we got home, Bea told the family about my fear, and the boys teased me. Bea's remarks were hard for me to understand, so I often withdrew when she was around. She told Shirley Jean to explain what a shadow was. Shirley Jean said she had seen her own shadow before but sometimes forgot, too.

I gradually learned the special meaning of weekends. Weekends meant visiting my grandparents in the country. Since Bea and Dad often worked weekends, they asked Shirley Jean to pack my things so I could stay with Grandma Mae and Grandpa. Weekends in the country became my idea of true peace. Everyone knew that when I was with my grandparents, I was not hiding behind a door—I felt safe.

YES, I'M THE GIRL BEHIND THE DOOR.

Although I remembered these visits as brief, Grandma Mae explained they often lasted weeks. The main reason for my stays was to give Shirley Jean a break from caring for the younger children.

Unlike me, my siblings showed little interest in visiting the country. The boys were deeply attached to the household, and their unpredictable temperament often frightened me. Bea's blunt and direct manner added to my discomfort.

Kathy, my older sister, occupied a unique place in the family. Though I was called "the baby," Kathy behaved more like one due to her dependence on Bea and her constant whining. Despite the labels, I felt older than her.

I kept my distance from Bea and the boys, finding comfort in quiet rather than their presence. Kathy sometimes joined me in the country and enjoyed playing the code word games—a tradition Grandma Mae had preserved since childhood.

Grandma Mae asked if we played code word games at home. I always answered honestly:

"No, ma'am, we only play when we're in the country or when Aunt Bobby Jean visits and Bea isn't around."

Grandma Mae smiled, recalling her own time spent with Aunt Bobby Jean, who was especially talented at creating and deciphering codes. Among all the games, Pig Latin was her favorite. Everyone laughed at the playful language, and even Grandpa joined in. Kathy was surprisingly good at the games. But when darkness fell, Kathy would whine. Grandma Mae and Grandpa did not like driving at night, and after one difficult trip, they told Dad they wouldn't bring Kathy home after dark anymore.

Mornings in the country arrived quietly. Grandma Mae always knew when I was awake. She prepared breakfast early, filling the kitchen with comforting aromas. As we ate, I asked if I could go on the swing afterward. Grandma Mae agreed, saying it would be warm enough to play outside.

I asked why there were two swings. Grandma explained that as the sun moved across the sky, the backyard would sometimes get too hot and other times the front yard would. This way, I always had a cool, shady place to play. Her simple wisdom made me feel understood.

One afternoon, while I was on the swing, Grandma Mae asked why I always hid behind the door at home. I didn't answer—just shrugged. She asked what I was afraid of and told me she and Grandpa noticed I was always behind the door during their visits, wondering if I was on punishment. Then she gently told me I didn't have to answer. She took my hand, brought me inside, helped me wash up, and offered me snacks.

Later, I told Grandma Mae and Grandpa about seeing something follow me and Bea in the sun. Bea said it was just my shadow, but when she told the family, the boys teased me. Grandma Mae listened kindly and told me Bea shouldn't have shared my fear with everyone.

She then asked if I remembered her explanation about the two swings. I repeated it, and both she and Grandpa applauded. Grandma then explained that just as the sun moves across the sky, shadows move too.

I wasn't sure how long I had stayed, but I knew Grandma Mae and Grandpa had recently taken me shopping for new clothes because the weather was getting colder. Grandma Mae said my fall clothes might not fit, reminding me that children grow quickly.

Grandma Mae moved around the kitchen with her usual care. I sat nearby, coloring in my new book—the one she bought on our shopping trip.

As I colored, Grandpa said he heard a truck. He looked out the window and saw Dad approaching. Grandma Mae insisted I finish breakfast before leaving. Dad joined us at the table.

Dad had exciting news: he planned to enter a contest in town before Christmas. Grandpa said he had read and heard about it.

During breakfast, Grandma Mae joked with Dad that I must have moved to the country since I had been staying so long. Laughing, she told him it was almost my birthday again. Their laughter filled the kitchen with warmth.

Dad and I left for home with hugs and kisses from Grandma Mae and Grandpa.

Grandma always reminded me to **use our secret code.**

Chapter 2: Twists & Secrets

This morning, sunlight filled the house as my brother David Lee left for work first. I went to my favorite place and waited until Dad and Bea woke up. Soon, I heard Dad coming to find me. He greeted me with a cheerful "Happy Birthday," his laughter echoing through the room as he pointed out that I was up even before the sun had risen, just like a little rooster, making me smile. Dad shared exciting news: my grandparents would be traveling from the country to join us in celebrating my birthday today.

Shirley Jean is a late sleeper; however, today she entered the room singing "Happy Birthday" to me. She paused and asked how old I was. I stretched out my hand, proudly holding up five fingers. She then asked me to count them, so I did: one, two, three, four, five—pausing at the last finger, happy that I remembered how to count and stopped right at age five.

I often did not see my sister Missie and my brother George in the mornings. They were always up early, eager to start their day, and would quickly head to their friends' homes. Being older, Missie and George had the freedom to come and go as they pleased. Their independence meant they could leave the house before the rest of us had even finished breakfast, and by the time our day was just beginning, Missie and George were already off enjoying their own activities. This early morning routine set them apart from the rest of us, who remained caught up in the hustle and bustle of the household.

Today, I saw and heard Kathy whining as usual, and the boys, meanwhile, were their usual lively selves, speaking loudly about something that captured their attention, although it felt as if no one else truly heard them except me.

Dad looked out the window and saw Uncle Cleo and Aunt Kutchie with their older girls. Bea and Dad went outside to greet them, engaging in extended exchanges, yet Uncle Cleo, Aunt Kutchie—Bea's sister—and the girls never came inside. This ritual unfolded each weekend as they prepared to head out for grocery shopping, a pattern that became as predictable as the sunrise, woven into the fabric of our family's weekly life. Bea and Dad went out shopping, taking my sister Kathy with them. Shirley Jean stayed home with me, getting me cleaned up and ready for my birthday.

Curious about our family's weekend rituals, I asked Shirley Jean why Dad and Bea always stood outside to talk with Aunt Kutchie and her family instead of inviting them inside. She told me, "You're growing up. Don't let Bea know you have those questions." Intrigued, she wondered aloud where that came from. I had heard my older siblings discussing this very thing—why our relatives never came inside the house—however, they were all remarkably close.

As we talked, Bea and Dad returned home, their arms full of grocery bags. I noticed that Kathy was not with them. While

Shirley Jean assisted with putting away the groceries, I heard a knock at the door.

Dad opened the door, and I heard a loud voice drawing our attention—it was how we always knew when Aunt Bobby Jean and Uncle CW had arrived; she was as loud as Bea. Soon afterward, Grandpa and Grandma Mae brought my favorite cake decorated with five bright candles, and Shirley Jean expressed her relief that she did not have to bake one herself this year. Everyone gathered together to sing "Happy Birthday" to me.

David Lee arrived home and handed me an ABC coloring book and a puzzle as birthday gifts. Bea gave me a beautiful Sunday school dress in my favorite color, which she called "banana yellow." My dad gave me a bank with money, which included money from Aunt Bobby Jean and Uncle CW to put into my bank.

Aunt Bobby Jean, who is Bea's sister, is well known in our family for her lively personality. Like Bea, she frequently uses the same expressions and carries herself with a certain familiarity. I often notice her clutching her purse, from which she occasionally pulls out a bottle and takes a drink. Her husband, Uncle CW, shares a similar habit, keeping his own bottle tucked away in his back pocket and drinking from it during their visits.

Whenever Aunt Bobby Jean and Uncle CW are together, their voices grow louder as they engage in animated conversations. If my brothers happen to be at home during these moments, the scene becomes even more boisterous, with the boys laughing at the exchanges between the adults.

Despite the cheerful atmosphere, I often feel uneasy around Aunt Bobby Jean, especially when Halloween approaches. She has a tradition of dressing up as a witch, painting her face black and wearing a costume that makes her look quite frightening. Her dramatic transformation during the holiday leaves an impression on me, and I find myself feeling afraid of her at those times.

She looked at me and asked, "When are you going to come out from behind that door?" Her question lingered, instantly catching the attention of everyone nearby. Grandma Mae, with her usual gentle manner, spoke up to comfort me. She reassured me that I could remain behind the door for as long as I needed if that was where I felt safe.

Aunt Bobby Jean, still unsatisfied, pressed further by asking, "Safe from who?" The question unsettled me, and I instinctively moved closer to my favorite hiding place, finding comfort in its familiar shelter.

Grandma Mae came over, greeting me with a warm hug and gentle kisses on my forehead. Before she left, she reminded me that Dad could bring me to the country when he was off work, giving me something to look forward to in the days ahead. Her affectionate farewell always made me feel special and cared for.

Dad understood the dynamic with Aunt Bobby Jean, knowing that she often claimed she was "just joking," even though her behavior made me uneasy. He was always aware of the effect she had on me, providing reassurance in his quiet way.

There was a knock at the door, and Dad opened it to reveal Aunt Janie standing beside my sister Kathy. As always, Kathy had her thumb in her mouth and was whining. Aunt Janie turned to Aunt Bobby Jean, urging her to calm down since her loud voice could be heard even from outside. In response, Aunt Bobby Jean began speaking in Pig Latin, directing her playful banter toward Janie and mimicking Kathy's whining. Aunt Janie told Aunt Bobby Jean she needed to stop drinking from that bottle, her words filling the room and capturing everyone's attention. Aunt Janie told Bea she would talk with her later.

The boys returned home and laughed at Aunt Bobby Jean's antics, always talking about her husband and calling him names. The boys found her very funny, joining in the lively atmosphere that always accompanied her visits.

Shirley Jean entered the room and asked me if this was my favorite cake that Grandma Mae had made for my fourth birthday. I said yes. She asked if we could have a piece of my cake. I said yes, and we went into the kitchen and had cake and ice cream. She then told me that for my next birthday, I would be six years old and in school, and I would have friends to invite over to celebrate. Curious, I asked Shirley Jean if she had friends when she was six. She explained that she did not have friends at that age, but she did have family—mostly cousins, who were all boys.

I admitted to Shirley Jean that I did not like boys, and she reassured me that it is common for little girls to feel that way since boys often play rough. However, she assured me that this would eventually change as I got older. Silently, in my mind, I thought, "No, it won't." That night, as I went to bed, my thoughts lingered on what it might feel like to have friends of my own.

This news brought both anticipation and uncertainty, hinting at the secrets and twists that lay ahead as I started a new chapter in my life. As I grew older, the contours of my world began to shift. Each twist and turn carried its own secret, shaping the path forward and offering glimpses of the changes yet to come.

It's Saturday morning. Bea is home, which is unusual. My siblings busied themselves with assigned chores, eager to finish so they could go outside. My responsibilities centered around keeping my favorite small place tidy, organizing puzzles, coloring books, and taking care of Sam. David Lee stopped by, as usual, to check on us while Bea and Dad were at work. Today, he was surprised to see Bea at home during lunch. David Lee engaged in conversation with Bea while picking me up and taking me to the window to observe the little girls playing outside.

"You are five years old and should be playing outside instead of playing behind the door alone. You should have friends," he said.

Bea asked David Lee why it bothered him, noting that it did not appear to bother anyone except him. David Lee never talked back to Bea; their conversation turned to what was for lunch and other chatter.

The barriers I felt were not just physical, like the door I sat behind, but also intangible currents of expectation winding through every corner of our home. I faded into the background, barely noticed, while the world moved on. I measured my time through daily routines and changing moods at home, as if my life were a clock.

One afternoon, I heard a strange noise coming from outside that startled me. Unsure and uneasy, I turned to Shirley Jean for an explanation, hoping she could help me understand what was happening. Shirley Jean calmly assured me that the noise was nothing new—it had always been there. Curious, I pressed her further, asking what the sound meant.

Shirley Jean's explanation of the siren noises left me feeling even more frightened. She told me that the sounds echoed through our neighborhood because there was a funeral home nearby, with casket boxes both in the front and the back of the building. The mention of casket boxes was confusing to me, and my uncertainty grew as I tried to understand what she meant. When I asked Shirley Jean what a casket box was, she simply replied that I did not need to know, warning that the knowledge would keep me from sleeping at night.

I confessed to Shirley Jean that I did not want to hear any more about it, admitting that the idea made me scared. She respected my feelings, and we left the conversation there, with my unease lingering in the quiet that followed.

Bea rarely invited me along when she ran errands around town; it was always my sister Kathy who accompanied her. On this particular day, however, Bea told me to put on my shoes because I would be joining her. The idea of going out with Bea did not appeal to me—I preferred to avoid outings altogether. Bea made her expectations clear: I was not to participate in her conversations with the other ladies. Instead, I was to remain quiet by her side, listening but staying silent as she talked with them.

Bea genuinely enjoyed chatting with the ladies outside, believing that these Southern visits were the foundation of long-lasting friendships. She often repeated this idea, though I did not fully understand what she meant.

On this occasion, as Bea and the ladies were talking, I overheard one of them telling Bea not to let me "put my eyes on them." I was not sure what that meant, and I felt uneasy, wondering if I had been disrespectful. Unsure, I looked down at the ground, trying to avoid drawing more attention to myself.

Later, on our way home, curiosity got the better of me, and I turned to Bea with a question that had been bothering me. I wanted to know why the ladies did not want me to look at them. Bea responded quietly, explaining that they were afraid of "the gift." I did not understand what that meant, so I pressed her further, asking what gift she meant. Bea's answer was, "I'll tell you when you're older."

When we returned home, I listened to the girls playing outside. I would quietly slip over to the window whenever I was alone in the front room, watching them closely. They were the same girls my brother David Lee had pointed out before. I started learning the lyrics to their songs, laughing along as I memorized each one. Whenever I had a moment to myself, I would sneak to the window and study how they played—drawing boxes in the dirt, tossing a rock, and jumping through the spaces, games that looked exciting to me.

One evening, Bea returned home from work and settled into her familiar routines. After changing clothes and refreshing herself, she joined Shirley Jean in the kitchen to help prepare supper.

I opened the door and sat on the steps, uncertain about whether I wanted anyone to notice me. From my quiet spot, I watched the girls outside as their lively songs and laughter drifted through the air. Their joyful energy drew me in, and I found myself captivated by the warmth and happiness of their play.

I overheard them mention that I was Mr. Coleman's daughter, Bunion. He was the only one who called me Bunion. At least to them, I was relieved that they did not know Bea, because she had a habit of giving us new names every day, some of which were not very flattering. It felt good to know they were not aware of that family quirk.

The girls invited me to join in their games. I confessed that I did not know how to play, but they were patient and took the time to show me the rules, guiding me step by step. Their kindness helped me relax, and soon I found myself genuinely enjoying their company. We laughed and played together, and when they asked if I wanted to be their friend, I happily said yes.

I heard Bea call out for me. I turned and saw her standing on the front step. Quickly saying goodbye to the girls, I hurried back home. As I reached Bea, she reminded me that I had gone outside without asking for permission. Unsure of how to respond, I listened quietly while Bea explained the importance of always asking before leaving the house. She told me I could not go into others' houses. Bea told me that I could play only in the front yard or on the porch. She instructed me to go into the house, clean up, and get ready for supper.

While I was preparing for supper, David Lee arrived home. I heard him call me "baby girl." Assuming he had a puzzle or coloring book for me, I approached him. He shared that he had driven by the house and seen me outside playing games with the girls. I laughed, and he smiled while expressing that he was happy I had gone out to play. I mentioned that I had made friends, and he responded by saying that he was proud of me. My friend's Portia Maria Stringer, Diana Maria Thomas,

I often found myself reflecting on my place within the family, wondering whether anyone truly noticed my tendency to withdraw or if my quietness had simply become an accepted part of the household's everyday rhythm. From my quiet spot in the house, I took careful stock of every detail—the sound of footsteps echoing across the floor, the hushed conversations exchanged between relatives, and the bursts of emotion that colored our days. These small moments, woven together, formed the backdrop of our daily life.

Before Bea left for work, I gathered the courage to ask her if I could go outside and play with my friends. This simple request marked a small but meaningful step, signaling my desire to be part of the world beyond my quiet observations. She said yes; however, I was not to go out until she let Shirley Jean know that she could watch me.

I finished breakfast and cleaned my area, then sat behind the door waiting to hear my friends. I told Shirley Jean that Bea said I could go out and play with my friends, and she laughed.

While I was outside enjoying the company of my friends, I suddenly heard a loud noise, referred to as a siren. Instantly, panic took over, and I ran as fast as I could across the yard. My knees ached painfully, the sensation of bone hitting bone urging me to hurry back to safety. The only thing on my mind was reaching my favorite spot inside the house, where I could sit and recover from the fright.

As soon as I entered the house, Shirley Jean noticed my arrival. She had also heard the piercing sound of the siren outside and, sensing my distress, was already making her way to find me. Her awareness and prompt action showed how attuned she was to both the environment and my emotional state. Without hesitation, Shirley Jean came to check on me, ready to offer comfort and reassurance after the startling noise.

She expressed her surprise that I had run off, especially now that I had friends, because she did not think I would be so quick to leave their company. Shirley Jean took a moment to explain that the siren was not meant for me or my friends, which was why the others had not run away. Her calm explanation helped ease my fears, and I began to understand that not every loud noise was a reason for me to panic or seek shelter. After she got me cleaned up and put oil on my knees, she asked if I wanted to join my friends again. I told her no, because they might laugh at me like the boys do. The sting of embarrassment lingered, making me reluctant to face my friends again so soon. Instead, I chose the comfort and safety of home, where I could quietly recover from both the fright and my sore knees.

I heard a gentle knock at the door. It was my friends, who had come to check on me. Their voices carried concern as they asked Shirley Jean if I was okay. They had not seen what had happened and were unsure why I had left so suddenly. From where I sat, I listened to Shirley Jean as she answered them.

As I sat inside, still shaken by the sudden noise, Shirley Jean came to check on me again. She calmly explained to both me and my friends that the loud sound we had heard was just a siren, and that it had startled us but was not a cause for concern. Her gentle reassurance helped my friends realize that the commotion was simply a reaction to an unexpected noise and not a sign of any real danger. With her soothing words, Shirley Jean eased the tension, making it clear to everyone that everything was fine.

She let the girls know that I would join them again tomorrow, and they nodded in understanding. Their kindness and acceptance, along with Shirley Jean's calm explanation, helped me feel more at ease, making it easier for me to look forward to playing with them again.

Chapter 3:
Contest of Endurance &
Holiday Triumph

As morning broke, I could hear the familiar voices and movement coming from the other room, signaling that Dad and Bea were already awake. From my usual spot, I quietly played with Sam, my loyal companion, while eagerly anticipating the possibility of spending time with my friend after abruptly leaving without saying goodbye.

Dad entered the room, knowing exactly where to find me, and asked if I wanted to accompany him to drop packages at my grandparents' home in the country. I agreed without hesitation, excited at the thought of seeing Grandma Mae and Grandpa. Before we left, Dad explained that I would not be spending the night and reminded me not to ask to stay, as he had many tasks to complete before Thanksgiving, the Christmas contest, and the holiday season. Understanding our visit would be brief, I quickly grabbed my doll Sam, and we set out for the country.

We arrived at my grandparents' house, and their warm welcome was unmistakable. Grandma greeted me with open arms, her laughter echoing through the rooms as she playfully teased me about having new friends. She joked that now that I had friends, I didn't come to visit as often. Her good-natured teasing brought smiles to everyone's faces.

Her joyful voice set a warm, cheerful tone for our visit, making it clear they were happy for me and proud of the steps I was taking to connect with others. I asked Grandma Mae and Grandpa if they would be coming to town for Thanksgiving this year. They explained that, with Dad being so busy preparing for the upcoming Christmas contest, they did not want to interrupt his schedule. We all laughed together, sharing in the excitement surrounding Dad's determination to win.

Dad reminded me that it was time to leave, noting that he and Uncle Cleo had a busy day ahead. As we prepared to go, Grandma Mae watched me and noticed something different. With a gentle smile, she pointed out that this was the first time I had visited without shedding tears when it was time to say goodbye.

Instead of sadness, I felt happiness and comfort—something Grandma Mae also recognized. She expressed her joy, saying she would cry happy tears now that I had begun making new friends. The change in my emotions was meaningful to her, marking a new chapter in my visits to their home. We shared hugs and kisses before heading back home.

After returning home and settling into my favorite place, I noticed Dad pacing the floor, his movements restless and purposeful. He answered the door, and Uncle Cleo entered, his familiar voice echoing through the entryway. More family members arrived than I had ever seen before, their presence replacing the peaceful atmosphere with lively conversation and movement. The change was unmistakable.

On Thanksgiving Eve, the house was alive with activity. Bea and Shirley Jean worked together in the kitchen, and the rich aromas of cooking spread through every room, signaling the start of the holiday festivities. Their movements were purposeful and familiar, filling the home with warmth and anticipation.

Thanksgiving Day was filled with memories of Madea. As family members visited, everyone seemed to reflect on Madea's absence. After the readiness of the Thanksgiving meal gave way to the holiday season, the focus gradually shifted toward the upcoming Christmas contest. Conversations began centering on the excitement surrounding the event. The contest became the main topic, overshadowing even the traditional celebrations. The anticipation grew stronger each day, and the household buzzed with discussions and preparations.

Excitement in the community was palpable, with talk of the event promising an extraordinary prize—a brand-new Ford truck.

The anticipation extended beyond our household and was evident everywhere. People discussed the contest with excitement, sharing predictions and stories. Family members, neighbors, and friends all seemed caught up in the buzz, and the shared enthusiasm brought people together.

I listened intently as Dad spoke about his determination to win. His confidence was obvious. Curious to understand more about how it worked, I asked Shirley Jean. She explained that Dad had officially entered the contest, and Uncle Cleo was there for support. This helped clear up my confusion, and I realized how significant the event was for our family.

We even visited the site in advance, where trucks were parked outside the Ford dealership and crowds had already begun to gather. The organizers announced that the contest would be held just before Christmas and that the winner would drive the new truck in the holiday parade. Dad seemed incredibly confident, celebrating as though he had already won.

After returning home and settling into my favorite spot, I heard activity outside. Looking out the window, I saw my friends gathering despite the chilly weather. Eager to join them, I asked Bea for permission. She reminded me of the cold and said I could play outside as long as I didn't go into anyone's house.

Bundled up in my coat, gloves, and hat, I stepped outside. Despite the chilly air, our spirits were high. During our conversation, one friend mentioned they hadn't seen me lately and assumed I must have been in the country. I explained that I had visited but couldn't stay because of the contest. My friends said their parents believed my dad would win. Their encouragement made me smile.

I told them that no one was talking about the holidays anymore—only the contest. The girls agreed the same was happening in their homes. The anticipation had overtaken the usual holiday excitement.

Dad told me I would be going to the country today because Shirley Jean wasn't available to babysit me. He explained I would spend the day with my grandparents. I was happy because Grandma Mae and Grandpa were always glad to have me visit. When we arrived, Grandma Mae helped me settle in while Dad said goodbye.

I'm not sure how long I stayed. One morning, Dad came to pick me up. Grandma Mae invited him inside while we finished breakfast. After gathering my things, we went to the kitchen, where she packed my favorite snacks and wrapped the rest of my cake. Dad needed to get ready for the contest and asked if they planned to come. Grandma Mae said they would be there for both the beginning and the end, but since it was too cold, they would only attend those key moments.

The family gathered to discuss the visiting time slots for everyone to show up—even though communication was limited to smiles and waves, or sometimes holding up words written on cardboard signs. I went with the family on the first day. It was early morning. Dad hugged and kissed everyone. The announcement stated that all contestants must be seated inside the truck immediately. Dad waved as he entered the truck with the big smile everyone knew him for. The contest had begun.

The weather played a major role, with some people choosing to stay and others leaving due to the cold. On the first day, everyone agreed the initial hours were the easiest. But by the next day, it became clear the real challenge was endurance. I heard people in the crowd say the contest would measure each contestant's determination and ability to endure hardship. The rules were strict, and Shirley Jean explained how they evaluated willpower and physical stamina.

Communication between participants was extremely limited— they relied on glances, smiles, or simple gestures. The silence added another layer of difficulty.

After the first night, several contestants withdrew. By the next morning, most participants had left. Only a handful remained by the second night. As the third morning arrived, and the evening approached, only three contestants were left, including my dad. Radio broadcasts announced that a winner would be determined that night and encouraged people to gather at the site.

Family members shared updates: only two contestants remained. My entire family gathered downtown for the final moments. I noticed Grandma Mae and Grandpa had come from the country despite usually avoiding night driving. Grandma Mae said the country would seem brighter tonight because of the excitement.

After what felt like an endless wait, the anticipation grew. Eventually, a door opened, and a man stepped forward to announce the results. The tension was unmistakable. Only one contestant remained.

As the contest drew to its dramatic conclusion, I found myself curious why Dad was still inside the truck. The silence and uncertainty made the moment feel longer. When the official stepped forward to make the announcement, we realized the strict rules required participants to stay inside until declared the winner.

I asked aloud why Dad hadn't gotten out. Uncle Cleo explained that Dad had to wait for the official announcement. Organizers then approached, opened Dad's door, and declared him the winner. Dad stepped out of the truck, greeted by enthusiastic cheers and shouts from our entire family.

Excitement filled the air as Dad was presented with the keys to a brand-new Ford truck. His heart was full of pride and joy. Our family returned home together to celebrate. The house filled with laughter, congratulations, and warmth.

I was happy to welcome my dad home. Although I assumed he would be exhausted and need rest, he was energetic, proud, and ready to prepare for the upcoming Christmas celebration. The family planned to participate in the Christmas parade. Even though the weather was freezing and the crowds were huge, everyone enjoyed the parade.

Chapter 4:
Sundays – Family and Faith

Sunday in our home always begins with a sense of peace and routine. Bea rises early, her voice filling the house as she sings "Amazing Grace." She and Shirley Jean work together in the kitchen, preparing the family's Sunday meal.

My siblings and I each have our own roles in the Sunday preparations. The girls are always the first to rise, making sure to bathe and dress for church before anyone else. After one group has finished preparing, the next group gets ready by bathing and changing into their church clothes in turn. Breakfast during these busy moments is a moving affair—each of us grabs something to eat as we go about our tasks, careful to keep an eye on the time so we are not late for Sunday school. Everyone works together, falling into a familiar routine that helps us start our Sunday with order and purpose.

Once everyone is ready, Bea gathers the boys and reminds them not to leave Kathy and me behind, knowing that we tend to move a bit slower. Although my knees feel better and I am walking faster these days, we all make it a point to leave the house together. As we set out, we meet up with our cousins and my sister Katie's children, who are close in age to Bea's children. I learned as I grew older that they are my nieces and nephews, which is why they call me "Aunt," joking along the way.

Each Sunday, our family follows a well-established path to Sunday school, enjoying the familiar routine and the company of one another as we walk. The boys in our family, who are uncles to my older sister Katie's children, share a special bond with their nieces and nephews. This dynamic brings a sense of togetherness that is especially noticeable during our Sunday traditions.

Family connections run deep—my mother, Bea, and Janie's mother, Aunt Kutchie, are sisters. Janie is my cousin, but out of respect for her upbringing by Madea, we acknowledge her as Aunt Janie and honor her wishes in this regard. These relationships are a source of strength and unity within our extended family.

I have observed that the boys behave differently when we are away from home, particularly appreciating the time spent with their nephews. My brothers do not spend time with the girls in the family, a trait that seems to have been passed down by our mother, Bea. Despite these differences, the sense of family remains strong, and we cherish the time we share as we make our way to Sunday school each week.

Our family always made a distinct impression with our sense of fashion when we attended church. We were known for dressing well and standing out among the congregation, each of us carefully choosing our outfits for Sunday services. However, Dad was the exception to this tradition. He had a particular fondness for vibrant colors and took a unique approach to dressing. Matching outfits or coordinating patterns did not concern him; instead, Dad viewed his shirt, pants, and jacket solely for their individual purpose, not for how they complemented each other.

Plaids with stripes, bold prints, or colorful shirts—Dad wore them all with confidence, never worrying about whether his clothes matched. His colorful and uncoordinated outfits became something of a signature look, setting him apart from the rest of us and adding a cheerful splash of personality to our family's presence at church. The family often found Dad's sense of clothing funny and full of humor. His disregard for conventional style norms and his bold choices were a source of amusement for everyone. Dad's outfits frequently sparked laughter and lighthearted comments among us, adding a playful element to our Sunday preparations and church gatherings. His cheerful attitude and the way he embraced his personal style made these moments memorable, reinforcing the warm and jovial atmosphere that characterized our family's time together.

Along the way, I often spotted my friends heading to their own church worship services, and we greeted each other with smiles and waves as we passed by.

Once our family arrived at church, we followed the usual routine by making our way downstairs to the basement, where Sunday school classes were held. These classes provided an opportunity for us to join other children in a smaller, more intimate group, allowing us to learn about scripture and deepen our understanding of biblical teachings before the main worship service began. The informal setting of Sunday school fostered meaningful conversations and helped us connect with our peers as we explored the lessons together.

After Sunday school concluded, we all gathered our belongings and moved upstairs to the sanctuary. There, the entire congregation came together to participate in the main worship service. This was a time for everyone to unite in praise, prayer, and reflection, creating a sense of togetherness.

Our family was quite large, and we filled seats in the sanctuary, often sitting together and making our presence known among the congregation. When the doors to the sanctuary opened, my father stood at the entrance in his role as the church's official greeter. He welcomed everyone with his characteristic warm, broad smile, guiding both members and visitors to their seats. My father knew everyone who attended, greeting them as friends and ensuring that everyone felt comfortable and included. Not all my siblings attended the service; two of them usually did not join us, though I was not sure of the reason.

After the church service concluded, our family returned home and exchanged our formal Sunday attire for comfortable clothes. This simple transition marked the beginning of our evening routine, where we all prepared to share the responsibilities of household chores. Bea led the way in the kitchen, carefully putting the final touches on dinner and ensuring everything was exactly right before the meal was served.

Once dinner was ready, each family member settled in at their own pace, creating a comfortable and relaxed atmosphere around the house. The conversation naturally shifted toward the pastor's message from earlier in the day. This shared time provided an opportunity for everyone to reflect together, discussing their thoughts and perspectives on the sermon.

Through these thoughtful exchanges, our family could connect on a deeper level. Each person was encouraged to consider the lessons and insights gained from the day's worship, fostering a sense of unity and understanding among us. The discussion not only allowed them to process their thoughts but also strengthened their knowledge. I listened and watched from behind the door.

These discussions often prompted my siblings to reach for their Bibles, eager to reflect on the scripture passages highlighted in the sermon. The exchange of insights quickly became a friendly competition, with each person keen to demonstrate their understanding of the Bible.

As the conversation unfolded, my brothers and Shirley Jean were particularly enthusiastic participants. Their commitment to reading the Bible from cover to cover set the tone for our evening gatherings. Each family member strove to show their depth of knowledge, referencing passages and sharing personal interpretations. This lively exchange not only encouraged thoughtful reflection but also fostered a sense of camaraderie rooted in faith and learning.

As evening settled and the house grew quiet, the family naturally gathered in the front room. This became a cherished time where each member could relax, setting aside the busyness of the day. The background noise of the television created a soothing environment for everyone to enjoy.

This peaceful routine marked the end of Sunday. It offered everyone the opportunity to unwind after a day filled with worship, family meals, and thoughtful conversation. By coming together in this way, we shared a sense of unity and contentment before heading off to rest for the night. I often wondered why it only happened on Sundays. It confused me.

I always bathed first, with Bea either helping me or allowing me to do it on my own. These moments alone with Bea were often accompanied by quiet conversations about faith and the importance of prayer. She shared her beliefs about God, emphasizing how significant prayer was in our lives.

During these talks, Bea explained that God chooses whom He wants to gift, and she encouraged me to think about the meaning behind this. I was always cautious when asking Bea questions, aware that her answers did not come with a gentle promise of explanation in the future. Whenever I asked what those gifts were, Bea simply responded that she would tell me once I was older. Her replies were always the same: "When you get older."

These conversations lingered with me long after they ended. Most nights, I drifted to sleep thinking about the gifts Bea mentioned, wondering what they might be and looking forward to the day when she would finally share more with me.

The morning after, Dad let me know that I would be going to the country that day, as Shirley Jean was not available to babysit me. He explained that I would spend the day with my grandparents, a prospect that always brought me joy. Grandma Mae and Grandpa were consistently happy to have me visit, and their warm welcome made me feel at home. Upon our arrival, Grandma Mae helped me settle in, ensuring I was comfortable, while Dad said goodbye before leaving for the day.

While settling in at my grandparents' house, Grandma Mae began asking about my friends and whether I had enjoyed Sunday school and the church service. I shared honestly with her, explaining that sometimes, during church, the ladies would run around the sanctuary, shouting and screaming. Bea was often among those women, and I admitted to Grandma Mae that seeing her behave that way made me feel sad.

I also told Grandma Mae that Bea only acted like that on Sundays. I asked about the words Bea used daily, except on Sundays. Grandma Mae asked me what words I had heard and who spoke them to me. As I began to repeat the words, Grandma Mae immediately stood up, visibly upset. She told me never to say those words again, explaining that they were curse words and questioning where I had learned them.

When I told her that Bea was the one who spoke those words and admitted that I did not know what they meant, Grandma Mae called for Grandpa and began to tell him the words I had repeated. Grandpa responded firmly, telling me that he did not want me to ever repeat those words again.

Grandma Mae gently asked if anyone else knew that I had used those words. I reassured her that only Shirley Jean was aware and explained that I had not repeated the words because Shirley Jean heard the same words that I did—Bea used them every day, which is how I remembered them. My curiosity was genuine; I just wanted to know what they meant.

When I approached Shirley Jean for an explanation, she told me that those words were curse words. I admitted to her that I did not know what they meant, and she warned me that if I ever repeated those words, Bea would spank me.

I told her that Bea started each morning—except Sundays— saying those words, which seemed wrong to me. I asked my grandparents not to tell Bea, because Bea said if I ever told them what happened at home, she would not allow me to visit them again. Grandma Mae suggested that Bea should consider managing my teen brothers in a comparable manner and then wondered aloud about my dad's opinion regarding Bea's choice of words. I shared with her that Bea often spoke harshly about Dad as well. Grandpa told Grandma Mae that she ought to discuss Bea's language, especially when it came to how she talked about their father in front of the children. Grandma Mae said she would talk to her son about why he let her speak to him that way in front of his kids.

During my stay at my grandparents' house, I found myself confiding in Grandma Mae about the troubling dynamics at home. She listened attentively as I shared my feelings about how Bea interacted with Dad, especially in front of us children. Grandma Mae expressed her concern, telling me that she would speak to her son about allowing Bea to speak to him in such a manner when his kids were present.

I also opened up to Grandma Mae about how Bea was fully aware of how much I understood about the family's affairs, frequently warning me not to reveal what went on at home. She insisted that I knew more than I let on and reminded me to keep this knowledge to myself. Grandma Mae said Bea was right—I knew more than I should. She told me I did not need to know what those words meant, nor care what they meant. "You are a child," she said, "and you must stay in a child's place." These conversations with Grandma Mae highlighted the complexities of trust and secrecy within our household, making me reflect on the expectations placed upon me and the importance of discretion that Bea emphasized.

From the expression on Grandma Mae's face, I could sense that I might be in trouble when I went home. I got quiet. Grandma Mae knew how to change the conversation by telling Grandpa that we could play Old Maid. It was a simple and fun game, and I always won—probably because Grandpa would lend me a hand. Somehow, Grandma Mae always seemed to end up with the queen, the Old Maid.

Grandma Mae called me into the kitchen, saying she had something she wanted to show me. When I got there, I saw that she had baked my favorite cake. We each had a slice together before deciding to play the code word game, a family favorite that could last all day. Grandpa joined in, and the afternoon was filled with laughter and friendly competition.

While I was settling in at my grandparents' house, Grandma Mae asked if I was ready for the first grade. I simply shrugged my shoulders, unable to give her a definite answer. My uncertainty showed that I was not sure how I felt about starting school. The thought of entering first grade brought mixed emotions, and I found it difficult to express how I truly felt.

As Grandma Mae's question lingered in the air, I found myself uncertain of how to respond. The silence was gentle, filled more with anticipation than discomfort. Grandpa soon joined the conversation, offering reassurance by comparing first grade to Sunday school, suggesting that I would have the chance to meet even more friends and enjoy new experiences, just as I had at Sunday school.

As Grandma Mae and Grandpa spoke with me, their gentle explanations provided comfort and clarity during a time of transition. Their reassuring manner made it easier for me to understand the changes happening around me, especially as I noticed how these shifts might affect Shirley Jean. Listening to their words, I felt a sense of sadness for Shirley Jean, who was getting ready to step away from her long-held role of caring for children. The prospect of this change weighed on me, as I recognized how much her presence had meant to our daily life and routines.

I trusted my grandparents enough to share my feelings openly. During our conversation, I admitted that the idea of starting school was beginning to feel less daunting. With their encouragement, I expressed both my hopes and uncertainties about attending first grade. Their support helped me process my emotions and look forward to the new experiences ahead, easing my worries and helping me feel more prepared for what was to come.

As summer approached, Grandma Mae gently encouraged me to prepare for the months ahead, reminding me that once school began, my attention would need to shift toward my studies. Her words were both a gentle nudge and a reminder of the changes soon to come.

Both Grandma Mae and Grandpa took the time to express their unwavering confidence in my abilities. They reassured me that they believed I would do well in school, voicing their trust in my capacity to adapt and succeed in an unfamiliar environment. Their supportive words provided me with a sense of comfort, easing my worries and helping me feel more prepared for the transition.

Their encouragement and faith in me offered reassurance as I started to look forward to the new experiences that awaited with the beginning of the school year. Knowing that I had their support made the prospect of starting school less daunting and filled me with hope for what was to come.

Grandma Mae let me know that my dad would not be picking me up that late. She thought he would come in the morning to get me. I mentioned to her that Dad had not brought my bag with him, but Grandma Mae just laughed. She reminded me that I always left clothes in the drawer at her house from previous visits. We both laughed as she teased me, saying I left clothes behind because I knew I would be coming back soon. The playful exchange brought us both joy, and with that, I took a bath and got ready for bed, feeling comforted by the familiar routine and Grandma Mae's warmth.

The next morning, Dad arrived to pick me up early because he had to go to work and would not be able to get me in the afternoon.

That morning, Dad mentioned he did not have time to sit down for breakfast. He assured me that Shirley Jean was at home and would prepare breakfast for me once we arrived. Before we left, Grandma Mae made sure to pack a plate for me to take along, carefully preparing my favorite foods. We shared a warm hug and a kiss before Dad and I headed out. As we drove away, we waved to Grandma Mae standing on the porch. She called out to Dad, reminding him not to speed on the road as we left for home.

Chapter 5:
The Womb of a Child

After Dad and I arrived home, he left almost immediately for work, leaving me with Shirley Jean. She kindly asked if I wanted breakfast, but I declined, remembering that Grandma Mae had already prepared breakfast and snacks for me to bring along. Even with food ready and available, I could not shake a strange and unfamiliar feeling. Though I knew I was not ill, I could not pinpoint the source of my discomfort.

As I listened to the voices of my friends outside, I recognized them but felt no desire to join them or go out and play. The usual excitement of gathering with others held no appeal for me. Instead, I retreated to my favorite spot in the house, seeking comfort in familiar surroundings. Feeling tired and out of sorts, I decided to take a nap, hoping rest might help me feel better.

Shirley Jean woke me, concerned and asking if I felt sick. I assured her I did not. Still, something felt off, and I struggled to find the energy to change my mood. When Bea arrived home, she told me to get up, take a bath, and head to bed if I was sleepy. She asked if I had slept at my grandparents' house the night before. I replied, "Yes, ma'am." The sense that something was wrong persisted—a feeling I often experienced when I was around my brothers Frank and Larry. Exhausted for reasons I could not explain, I prepared for bed, hoping rest would help me feel better.

It was morning, and I noticed the sunrise looked different here than it did at my grandparents' place in the countryside. While Bea moved around, I observed my father leaving for work as I sat in my usual spot. I listened to Bea tell Shirley Jean that school would start soon. She mentioned she had checked with the school to see if my birthday would allow me to begin first grade—even though I would turn six on November tenth—and they told Bea I could begin in September. This meant it would be Shirley Jean's last summer babysitting. I remained uncertain of the exact date I would begin school; the uncertainty lingered in the back of my mind as the household settled into its usual rhythms.

That morning, my teenage brothers Frank and Larry decided to stay at home instead of going out with their friends. It was not unusual for them to change routines. One of my older brothers, Lewis—who often alternated between staying in and going out— also chose to spend the morning at home.

As was common, my sister Missie and my brother George did not participate in the games played at home. They typically left the house to join their friends, choosing to spend their time outside rather than engaging in family activities.

The games played at home usually involved cards, questions about literature, and a significant amount of Bible trivia, reflecting the household's familiarity with scripture and biblical stories.

During these trivia sessions, my siblings actively participated. They checked their Bibles to verify answers and maintain fairness. Familiarity with a balanced selection of Bible verses among all participants contributed to a calm and enjoyable experience, with everyone feeling comfortable and engaged.

Card games in our household were often a source of excitement and energy. Sessions frequently became lively, with voices raised in arguments and the atmosphere charged by the spirit of competition.

At the card table, Shirley Jean stood out as a formidable competitor. She played each game with remarkable skill and determination, rarely losing and consistently claiming victory. Her winning streak became a point of pride in the family, and it was well known that defeating her was a rare achievement. My brothers seldom managed to outplay her, which only heightened the sense of rivalry and excitement that surrounded each session.

Among my siblings, my brother Lewis—affectionately called Baby Boy—stood out as the youngest of Bea's older children. Lewis was known for his curiosity and enthusiasm, especially about the Bible and the English language. He frequently corrected others' grammar and word usage, which sometimes caused friction among family members, despite the occasional annoyance.

My teenage brothers had a reputation for troublesome behavior that was evident to anyone observing them. Their actions and attitudes made it clear why most people, including myself, preferred not to spend time around them. Shirley Jean, along with everyone else in the house, understood that I was genuinely afraid of my brothers, and this fear was well known within our family.

On this day, there was a higher level of household activity than usual. From my place behind the door, I watched one of my teenage brothers display obvious signs of distress. The tension was palpable, and the atmosphere felt different from other days.

Adding to the charged environment, my sister's loud boasting further irritated the teenage boys. Her excitement and energy clashed with their mood, intensifying their annoyance and contributing to the overall sense of unease in the house.

My body lurched forward toward the wall, unsettled by the commotion unfolding nearby. From my vantage point behind the door, I watched anxiously as one of my brothers paced back and forth, his agitation evident in the way he spoke loudly to himself. I saw him kick the wall with force and strike the table, each action increasing the tension in the room. Remaining hidden behind the door after picking myself up from the floor, I waited patiently for him to move away, hoping for a chance to reach Shirley Jean for safety.

I watched as my brother approached the front door, prompting me to move quickly behind Shirley Jean's chair. Shirley Jean was laughing and making remarks, clapping her hands in celebration—something I often joined in during her victories. I responded in the usual way, participating in her enjoyment.

Meanwhile, my brother paced across the floor, speaking loudly. I hesitated to move, uncertain about returning to my usual spot behind the door, but chose to remain where I was, gripping Shirley Jean's chair tightly. I deliberately avoided eye contact with my brother as his anger grew and he drew closer to Shirley Jean.

I felt reassured knowing my brother would avoid any direct conflict with Shirley Jean. In our household, my brothers often called her "Hulk," a nickname that captured her formidable presence and their belief that she could stand up to any of them. Because of this reputation, the likelihood of my brother confronting her seemed low even during tense moments.

From my position, I watched my brother walk past the dining area, leading to the kitchen where our card games often took place. I assumed he was heading toward the kitchen to distance himself from the tension. Meanwhile, I stood quietly behind Shirley Jean's chair, waiting for him to pass. My plan was to return to my original spot once he left, but the uneasy atmosphere made me hesitate.

For a moment, everything in the room grew still, the tension lingering in the air. Suddenly, the quiet was disrupted as I collapsed to the floor behind Shirley Jean's chair, overcome by pain and fear, screaming in shock.

The pain I experienced was indescribable and overwhelming. Shirley Jean regularly instructed me not to cry, but I was unable to speak and could only express myself through screaming. After the incident, I noticed blood running down my legs, and as the bleeding intensified, panic and confusion filled the room.

Finally, Shirley Jean stood up, leaned down to pick me up, and saw the blood running down my legs onto the floor. Alarmed, she urgently yelled for someone to call emergency medical services. "She is bleeding!" she exclaimed. Shirley Jean grabbed towels, packing them around me, and tried desperately to stop the bleeding while holding me tightly. Hearing her shouting for an ambulance heightened my panic, confirming how serious the situation was.

Everyone in the family gathered on the front porch, watching and waiting for the ambulance. Shirley Jean carried me outside, and I clung to her desperately, hoping she would not let go. My pain felt unexplainable—something only God could understand. Shirley Jean paced up and down the street while I screamed, and people asked what was wrong. She only replied that the ambulance was on the way.

David Lee, who checked on us frequently, arrived while Shirley Jean was walking with me in her arms. He asked what had happened, and Shirley Jean said that one of my teenage brothers had kicked me. David Lee immediately told her, "Get in the car. I'll drive her to the hospital—let's go." He called out the car window, telling my brother—the one who had kicked me—to leave and not return until he came back from the hospital.

David Lee made sure neither Dad nor Bea would arrive home unless someone was present to ensure my brother's safety. When we reached the emergency room, David Lee rushed inside to get help while Shirley Jean held me tightly as she exited the car. The commotion inside the hospital was immediate—voices surrounded us, asking, "What happened? Where is the blood coming from?"

Shirley Jean tried explaining the situation as the hospital staff attempted to take me from her arms. I clung tightly to her, unable to let go. The chaos and noise in the room felt overwhelming, and my fear grew. My screams became louder, and someone asked how old I was. Despite Shirley Jean's attempts to comfort me, my distress continued.

As the chaos continued, the doctor approached and told Shirley Jean he needed to examine me to find the source of the bleeding. His tone was calm yet urgent, emphasizing the need for immediate medical attention. Though I was hesitant, the doctor's reassurance made it clear that the exam was necessary for my well-being.

With the nurses assisting, the doctor began assessing the injury to locate and stop the bleeding. His urgency reflected the seriousness of the situation. Throughout the examination, Shirley Jean stayed close, offering comfort as the medical team worked quickly.

I felt a prick in my arm and yelled in pain. The doctor explained it was something to help me relax while they figured out what was wrong. I heard everything but could not respond; there was no more pain after the medicine took effect. The doctor spoke gently as he dried my tears. Shirley Jean said, "Dr. Burnham delivers you—remember, I take you to his office for your visits." He remarked that I was familiar with him; although I did not speak, I recognized him from earlier visits. He noted I was becoming a "big girl."

When the procedure was complete, Bea entered the room as the doctor applied gauze to cover and secure the wound. The doctor explained the procedure to Bea and Shirley Jean, telling them that stitches had been required to close the wound. He also gave instructions for daily care and healing. A nurse prepared a bag of supplies.

I listened as the doctor instructed us to keep the area clean and to contact the office or return to the hospital if any issues arose. He asked for an office visit in two weeks to check the healing and determine if the stitches should be removed. He warned that I should not play outside. He laughed lightly, saying he often saw me behind the door instead. Shirley Jean added, "She has friends now. I've never seen her without her doll." Dr. Burnham handed me a small bag of candies before leaving, saying, "Go home and check on your doll—I know she misses you."

On the ride home, Bea and my brother sat in the front seat while Shirley Jean held me in the back. Shirley Jean asked Bea if she had noticed the nurse with a bandage on her nose. Bea said she had. Shirley Jean explained that during the struggle at the hospital, when the nurse tried to restrain me, I had bitten her nose. She added that she refused help, and the nurse ended up injured.

At that moment, I became aware of feeling unwell and began to cry. Shirley Jean said my reaction was understandable considering how long I had been screaming. No one had been able to approach me or calm me until I was given the injection. Bea asked what had happened, and Shirley Jean explained that my brother had kicked me, causing the entire incident.

When Bea asked for clarity, Shirley Jean said that she and my brothers had been playing cards. After losing, my brother Frank became upset and kicked her. Bea pointed out that I had not been part of the game and questioned why he had directed his anger toward me. She raised her voice, asking where my brother was.

Shirley Jean told her that David Lee had instructed my brother to leave the house until everyone returned from the hospital. I felt uneasy, sensing that Bea and Dad might be too harsh on my brother.

After returning home, I spoke only with Shirley Jean, who cleaned and changed my bandage. Each time she tended to the wound, I felt helpless and embarrassed. The discomfort was difficult, even when using the bathroom. The treatments involved creams and antibiotics, and a burning sensation often followed each bandage change. Healing felt endless.

I have ongoing concerns about my safety due to my brother's past actions. Despite seeing him daily, I cannot find comfort when he is nearby. This fear separates me from the rest of the household. I feel isolated and disconnected, unable to reconcile my feelings with those around me.

I found myself longing for Bea's guidance to help me make sense of everything. There was so much confusion, and I struggled to find words to describe what had happened. No one in the family discussed the incident, nor offered explanations. It seemed forgotten, while my doubts remained unresolved. I hoped Bea could help me understand.

Bea often said I was wise beyond my years, possessing a perspective others did not recognize. At present, the only life altered by these events was my own. The weight of my emotions was overwhelming. Each night, I fell asleep with the curtain slightly open so I could see the stars, dreaming of adulthood and leaving everything behind. It became a routine comfort, offering solace in uncertainty.

Later, I returned to Dr. Burnham's office for a follow-up visit. Shirley Jean accompanied me, as Bea was working. The nurse helped me change and assisted me onto the bed. After examining the area, Dr. Burnham said he recommended leaving the stitches in for one more week. He gave me candy and said he would see me again in a week, praising how well I had kept the wound clean.

After a week passed, Shirley Jean told me it was time for another appointment. David Lee drove us. Dr. Burnham examined the wound, pleased with how well it had healed. A nurse applied numbing cream, telling us it would take about fifteen minutes before the stitches could be removed. Dr. Burnham gave me a piece of candy and promised I'd get it back after the cream worked.

He removed the stitches, telling me to alert him if I felt discomfort. I said no throughout the procedure. He said the outcome was good and reminded me to continue applying the cream throughout the day, especially after using the restroom. Afterward, he asked to speak with us in his office.

Shirley Jean helped me dress, and we went to his office. He greeted us warmly and asked whether anyone had spoken to me about the incident. Shirley Jean said she was unsure. His concern for my emotional well-being was clear.

Dr. Burnham emphasized the importance of giving me a safe space to express my thoughts and feelings. He wanted me to have the chance to talk about what happened and gain understanding. He explained that if discussing it was uncomfortable, he could recommend someone experienced to speak with us. He asked Shirley Jean to have Bea contact him.

Shirley Jean mentioned that I was preparing for school soon. Dr. Burnham asked me how I felt about starting first grade. I shrugged, and when he clarified, I said yes—it made me uneasy.

He gently asked me what had happened. I said, "My brother kicked me." He asked, "How do you feel about that?" I replied, "It makes me sad." The question overwhelmed me, and I began to cry.

Dr. Burnham comforted me, saying it was okay to cry and that expressing my feelings would help. This was the first time someone openly accepted my tears. His reassurance helped me feel understood and safe. He asked that I return in two weeks and said he would arrange for someone who works with children to talk to me, and for Bea or Shirley Jean to meet with a specialist as well.

While we waited for David Lee to return, Shirley Jean shared that Dr. Burnham was the doctor who had delivered Bea's only child in the hospital—me. Curious, I asked what a midwife was. Shirley Jean explained that a midwife is a woman who helps mothers give birth at home. This helped me understand what made my birth different from the rest of my siblings.

Once we got home, I struggled with thoughts and emotions I could not express. Shirley Jean helped me prepare for a nap. When Bea returned from work, Shirley Jean told her about Dr. Burnham's recommendations. Bea said another doctor's visit was unnecessary, believing I no longer had issues.

Even now, I continue to struggle with uncertainty about the changes in my life. This doubt weighs on me, bringing a deep sense of embarrassment. These feelings make me withdraw from attention, leading me to seek comfort in my safe place.

Instead of joining my friends, I remain indoors where I feel more in control. I spend time arranging my doll and puzzles. The simple act of organizing brings me comfort, easing my mind.

My sense of safety is strongest when I am behind the door, separated from the rest of the household. This physical boundary gives me security. I avoid interactions with my teenage brothers, around whom I feel especially uneasy. Their presence is intimidating, so I stay out of their way.

Reflecting on that day I returned from my grandparents', I remember the overwhelming urge to retreat to my safe place. Instead of playing with my friends, I stayed behind the door, seeking protection from the uncertainty around me. I could not explain the feelings driving my actions or understand what was happening inside me. I simply could not express my emotions in a way others could understand.

Chapter 6:
Navigating First Grade — Facing Fears and Finding Resilience

After a return visit to Dr. Burnham's office, he arranged for me to speak with a counselor and assured Bea that he felt it would be beneficial for me as the time to start first grade approached. There was a noticeable shift in the household. I was scheduled to meet with a counselor two days a week, which meant Shirley Jean would be taking me to these visits. Everyone seemed focused on getting ready for this new chapter, treating it as an important event. Amid this preparation, I found myself wondering if anyone else in the family had ever actually attended first grade before. This thought lingered in my mind as we moved through the routines leading up to the start of school, adding to my uncertainty about what to expect.

Bea took me shopping for school supplies, even though I did not understand why she was buying these things. I was not planning to go to school, so the purpose behind the shopping trip was confusing to me. During this time, Bea spoke to me about starting first grade as if it were something unfamiliar to everyone in our family. It felt as though no one had ever experienced first grade before, which only added to my uncertainty.

As September arrived and my birthday approached in November, I noticed that Bea repeated the same words about school every day. I mentioned this to Shirley Jean, explaining that Bea's daily reminders did not make sense to me. The repetition left me puzzled, and I struggled to understand why Bea felt the need to say the same things day after day. Shirley Jean said she had no idea.

On Sunday night, Bea announced that it was time for bed, reminding me that tomorrow would be my first day of school. The night felt impossibly long as I lay awake, unable to find rest. I do not recall falling asleep at all; morning seemed to arrive suddenly, marked by Bea waking me and insisting I get ready so I would not be late for my first day. This was unfamiliar territory for me—no one had ever needed to wake me before. Usually, I was the first to rise, just as Dad always said, "like the rooster."

As Bea moved through the morning routine, she spoke about everything except the recent events that continued to weigh on me. Everyone behaved as though nothing had happened, carrying on with their regular tasks and conversations. While Bea prepared my lunch, she noticed my tears and asked why I was crying, pointing out all the snacks she had packed for me. Despite her attempts to reassure me, I was afraid the children at school would ask questions about what I had been through. I did not feel ready to face them or the uncertainties of the day ahead, and it seemed that Bea did not truly understand how I felt.

As we left the house, I found myself surrounded by a crowd of children and parents, all moving purposefully toward the school. The sight was overwhelming, and my thoughts were consumed by how I might find my way back home, especially since the school was not far away.

I remembered Shirley Jean's advice from our trips downtown. She had taught me the importance of picking out a landmark—something distinct that could guide me if I ever got lost. I looked around, searching for anything that stood out, hoping to imprint it in my mind as a reference point for returning home.

While Bea spoke with other parents, she pointed out children from Sunday school, suggesting I might talk to them. Her efforts seemed aimed at helping me feel more comfortable, but my focus remained on the idea of safety and finding my way back should I need to.

Bea told me to get in line with the other kids to enter the classroom. Once inside, I saw the same boys who had teased me in the yard over the summer when I was playing with my friends. I chose a desk far away from them.

As soon as the teacher stepped out of the classroom, the same boys who had teased me before began to target me again. They called me names like "skinny," "broomstick," and "wiener up your butt," referencing my brother's habit of kicking what they called "pies" onto me. Their words were cruel, and I could hear other children laughing along, which made the experience even more humiliating and painful.

Unable to cope with the overwhelming emotions, I stood up, grabbed my lunch bucket, and ran out of the school, heading home with tears streaming down my face. The laughter and taunts echoed in my mind as I hurried away, desperate for the comfort and safety of my favorite place behind the door with Sam, my puzzle, and coloring books. I did not want the outside world.

When I arrived at the house, Bea opened the door and immediately questioned me: "Why did you leave school?" Overcome with emotion, I could not stop crying. Through my tears, I tried to explain that I did not understand what had happened to me at school. The other children laughed at me and called me names I did not even know the meaning of. Bea, however, did not listen to my explanation. Instead, she spanked me and walked me back to school. This happened repeatedly.

After these emotional experiences at school, Dad sat me down for a serious talk. He told me firmly, "When your mother takes you to school, you better not leave." His tone made it clear that he meant every word; I had never heard him speak to me like that before, and I understood the importance of what he was saying.

Bea took me back to school one last time, making sure I knew I had no choice in the matter. She wanted to ensure I understood that I needed to stay and not leave again. That day, the girls I had met in the front yard came over and sat beside me in class. From that moment on, we became close friends—sitting together during lessons and lunch, and walking home together every day.

On Mondays and Fridays, Shirley Jean would always wait for me at school so she could take me to my appointment. These appointments were for me to visit my counselor. With Shirley Jean by my side, I felt a little more at ease about having to go. Her presence made the experience more manageable, and I appreciated having someone familiar to accompany me each week.

After attending a few sessions with my counselor, I eventually reached a point where I was able to speak with her alone, without anyone else accompanying me. This new independence gave me a sense of confidence and control over my own healing process.

Shirley Jean was excited about this change as well. She looked forward to having time to herself in the waiting area, often bringing her book to read while I attended my sessions. I told my friends that I needed to visit my counselor, which was why I was unable to play with them on Mondays and Fridays in the evenings. My friends listened and seemed to understand, accepting my reason for missing out on our usual activities together.

It was my birthday, and I had just turned six years old. In many ways, I felt older than my age, shaped by the experiences I had already faced. Earlier that day, Dad encouraged me to let my friends know about the birthday party he had planned for me after school. As I walked over to the girls, I shared the news that Dad said I was having a party and asked if they would come. Both girls happily agreed.

After school, my friends changed into clothes for the celebration and came over to my house. We played games together, filling the afternoon with laughter and fun. Dad had cake and ice cream for us, making it a special treat. This birthday was my first without Grandma Mae and her husband, Grandpa, but their absence was softened by the presence of my friends and the joy we shared. The celebration marked a new chapter for me, surrounded by friendship and the warmth of my dad's caring spirit.

We had so much fun with Dad during my birthday celebration. I had always known him to be full of laughter, and that day was no different. We played games together, and Dad entertained us by singing all the songs he had made up. My friends loved Dad's songs; we all laughed at the funny lyrics and the joy he brought to the party. After singing "Happy Birthday," we enjoyed cake and ice cream. When the party was over, Dad and I walked my friends home, which was only a block away.

On the way home, his laughter echoed the joy we had shared during the celebration, and I felt comforted by his presence. Walking together reminded me how much my friends enjoyed Dad's playful spirit and the songs he made up for us. After a day filled with friendship and happiness, being with Dad made the walk home feel safe and warm—a moment I cherished after all the excitement of my birthday party.

After Dad and I arrived home, Bea told me to take a bath and go to bed. "You have school in the morning," she said. While I was in the bath, I could hear Bea screaming and cursing at Dad about the bottle in his back pocket. I did not know why that bottle bothered her. The noise in the house bothered me. I finished and went to bed as Bea had said. I could still hear Bea cursing angry words about that bottle.

I got out of bed and went to the front room to sit behind the door as usual. I had always felt a need to be close to Dad when Bea was angry.

After what seemed to be the longest time, Bea ordered me back to bed. As she walked with me, she told me, "Your dad is deaf." I did not know what that meant. Bea said, "He is hard of hearing." I thought to myself, *Dad cannot hear? Then how does he answer me when I talk to him?* It was hard to sleep in this house. I pulled the curtain back so I could see the stars and fell asleep dreaming of an unknown place.

I woke up early, eager for another day at school and the chance to see my friends again. As soon as I arrived, they greeted me with enthusiasm, clearly happy to see me too. The girls immediately started sharing stories about how much they had enjoyed my dad's playful spirit, remarking on how funny he was and how he always came up with silly songs. Hearing them talk about my dad this way made me smile, as it was exactly how I knew him—always cheerful, making up songs, and bringing joy wherever he went.

I did not tell them what happened after they left, nor what Bea said. Not one thing about Dad being deaf. I was still talking to Dad, and he listened to me. I did not want to hear Bea's mouth and all that cursing. I started spending more time at my friends' house.

After school, one of my friends' moms began talking with us about becoming Brownies, explaining what an adventure it would be—camping, field trips to the zoo and Six Flags in Memphis, pajama parties, learning how to bake cakes, selling Girl Scout cookies, Saturday afternoon meetings, traveling and meeting other groups from different areas. It sounded like fun, and we said yes.

One of my friends' moms asked Bea if I could join. I could not believe she said yes. Now I was out of the house—sleepovers, camping, field trips—it felt good to have friends. The noise at home seemed to never go away. I noticed things about Dad and that bottle. Dad was not in the house as much. I did not know where he was going. Bea screamed at him often, and I would feel sad for him.

I began to speak with my counselor about Bea saying my dad was deaf and what it truly meant. I shared the experiences I had following my birthday, including the confusing things Bea said. Having conversations with my counselor became an important way for me to process the emotions and events I experienced at home. These discussions provided me with the opportunity to reflect on my family dynamics and gain a clearer understanding of my own feelings and reactions.

During my sessions, my counselor explained that when a person is truly deaf, they are unable to hear what others say. I responded by sharing that my dad did, in fact, hear me and answer when I spoke to him. The counselor advised that if my dad continued to communicate with me and did not show signs of not responding, I should feel comfortable continuing to talk to him. I felt a sense of relief after my visit.

After Shirley Jean and I arrived home, I knew I needed to complete my homework before anything else. I focused on my assignments, determined to finish them before dinner and my evening bath. Once my homework was done, I bathed, ate supper, and settled into my favorite spot to relax for the night.

While I was unwinding, I overheard Bea talking loudly in the next room. She repeated, as she often did, that she had never had a drink in her life and had never gone to a club or even attended a house party. Despite these claims, Bea frequently left out the part about her cursing, which she did regularly— "cursing like a sailor," as people say. My friends and I found it to be just a term people used for repeating strong language daily.

Dad managed to do well for a short period, but inevitably he returned to his old habits. Bea, growing increasingly weary of this pattern, expressed her frustration openly. She said she was tired of dealing with the situation and that her patience had worn thin. I, too, found myself exhausted—not just by Dad's actions, but by Bea's constant yelling that filled our home with tension.

During one particularly heated exchange, I overheard Bea telling Dad to go live with his girlfriend. Her statement made it clear that she was no longer willing to tolerate his behavior and underscored the ongoing strain within our household. The emotions in the room were intense, with tempers frequently flaring and little resolution in sight. Bea's words revealed the depth of her frustration and the instability that continued to affect our family.

After witnessing these confrontations, I sought support from my counselor. During our session, I explained that no one seemed to have answers for me, and that the issues at home always seemed to revolve around Bea, Dad, the bottle, and now the mention of Dad's girlfriend. These topics created a sense of confusion and uncertainty, leaving me searching for clarity and understanding amid the ongoing turmoil. My counselor offered a space for me to share my experiences and emotions, helping me process the challenges I faced within my family.

I asked Shirley Jean why everyone screamed in our house. "When I visit my friends' homes, no one is screaming," I told her. Shirley Jean responded that Dad had a hearing problem and sometimes read lips. "That's what Bea says," she added. "He doesn't want to hear Bea's mouth. Not only does he hear you, he answers you."

I began going to bed with tissues in my ears so that I could not hear what anyone said. I looked out the window at the stars until I fell asleep.

Even so, I continued to listen and observe the interactions within my home, striving to make sense of the environment and the behaviors I witnessed. This approach allowed me to learn from those around me while maintaining my own boundaries and avoiding unnecessary trouble.

I went to visit my counselor and discussed how I felt about what happened to me not being acknowledged. It seemed as if everyone had moved on, as if it never happened. The house was full of people moving around, avoiding one another and not responding.

As time passed, I found myself increasingly drawn to spending time at my friends' house. The environment there offered a sense of comfort and relief that I could not find at home, where tension seemed to linger constantly. My visits became a much-needed escape from the undercurrent of stress that defined my everyday life with family.

Bea made it clear that she had never consumed alcohol or attended clubs or parties, emphasizing her own standards. Nevertheless, her emotional responses were frequently characterized by language that I found overly intense and unsettling. After noticing how frequently Bea used such words, I asked Shirley Jean for clarification about this behavior.

Shirley Jean took the time to explain to me why it was important to avoid using certain words that I had heard during arguments at home. She stated plainly that these words were not suitable for children, even if adults used them when frustrated.

One afternoon, after the school day had ended and my classmates had been dismissed, my teacher asked me to remain in the classroom. I stayed seated at my desk, listening as the sounds in the hallway faded and the room became quiet and still. When everyone else had gone, she called me to her desk. With a gentle but serious tone, she began our conversation by asking if I knew why she had asked me to stay behind. Unsure of her reasons, I could only shrug my shoulders, unable to offer an explanation.

During our conversation, my teacher said she had observed a noticeable decline in my participation in class. She pointed out that my attention span seemed to have changed compared to earlier in the year. Her approach was gentle and caring, making it clear that her concern was genuine and that she wanted to understand the reasons behind my shift in behavior and engagement with schoolwork.

She told me she would be sending a note home to my mother. The note would address her observations about my lack of attention in class and her belief that I might not be getting enough sleep, which could be causing me to nod off during lessons. She asked if I had any questions. I said, "No, ma'am." She said I could go home and that she would see me tomorrow.

I walked out the door and saw my friends waiting down the hallway for me. They asked what had happened and why I had been asked to stay behind when I had been doing well. I told them I had not been paying attention in class and that it was a warning that I could do better. I told them she had given me a note to give to Bea, meaning I would not see them for a while because I was going to be punished. My friends said, "It's okay, you can do it, because we still have time before school is out for the summer."

Shirley Jean reminded me about the conversation with Dr. Burnham and my counselor, who both believed that I should not attend school until the following year due to the challenges I had experienced over the summer. She reassured me that it was fine and told me she would speak with Bea to explain the situation. Shirley Jean then asked if I wanted to stay home and begin school next year. Overcome with emotion, I began to cry and insisted that I wanted to continue with my schoolwork. I explained that it was not uncommon for children to receive notes from teachers and that others had gone through similar experiences and improved.

Shirley Jean encouraged me, reminding me that there was still enough time for me to improve my grades. She offered to study with me, and her reassurance and willingness to help gave me hope that I could overcome my difficulties and do better in school.

When I showed her my homework, she looked at it and asked, "What?" I didn't respond. She insisted, "No, you're going to do your homework and start going to bed early." She emphasized that I needed to know the answers to these questions before going to school, reinforcing her belief that I already knew the answers and simply needed to apply myself.

When Bea arrived home, she immediately asked why I was not outside playing with my friends and was instead sitting quietly behind the door. Shirley Jean stepped in, explaining to Bea about the note I had brought home from my teacher. She made it clear to Bea that, because of the teacher's concerns, I would not be allowed to attend Girl Scout meetings or go out to play until my grades improved.

Shirley Jean also commented that she had reviewed my homework and believed I already knew the answers before I even began school. This emphasized her belief that my struggles were not due to a lack of ability, but perhaps something else. Bea responded with confidence in my abilities, stating that I knew more than just what was taught at school.

Shirley Jean asked Bea if she wanted me to stay out of school for the rest of the year and start over the following year. Bea was adamant in her response, saying, "Hell no, she's going to school and getting back to where she was when she started." This exchange made it clear that both Bea and Shirley Jean held high expectations for me and were determined that I would overcome these challenges and return to my previous level of success in school. I finished my homework, ate supper, took a bath, and went to bed—and this became a routine.

During one of my regular visits to my counselor, she acknowledged that I was continuing to complete my schoolwork. She expressed concern that the disciplinary measures at home might be a bit harsh, especially considering the challenges I had faced before the school year began. Wanting to understand how I was coping, she mentioned that she had already spoken with my teacher regarding my performance. My teacher had reported that I was doing well at first, which prompted my counselor to ask what had caused my performance to decline after such a promising start, especially since both she and Dr. Burnham had previously recommended that I take time off during my first school year.

In our conversation, I shared that I sometimes fell asleep in class. My counselor encouraged me to try going to bed earlier to help with my focus and participation. I agreed, responding respectfully, "Yes, ma'am."

After spending more time at home, I dedicated myself to focusing on my schoolwork and paid closer attention during lessons. I became more engaged in class activities, making a consistent effort to participate and improve. My hard work did not go unnoticed. Before long, my teacher observed positive changes in my behavior and academic performance. She recognized my improvement and, one afternoon, asked me to stay after school again.

That day, rather than feeling anxious, I felt a sense of accomplishment as she handed me a note to take home to my mother. This note recognized my progress and confirmed that I was back on track and on my way to advancing to second grade. Feeling proud of how far I had come, I chose not to wait for my usual ride home with my friends. Instead, I walked with other children who lived near my home, carrying with me a sense of achievement and hope for the future.

Chapter 7:
Family, Loss & Growth

During the summer, everything seemed to be going well. I found joy in my time as a Girl Scout, and our meetings took place on Saturdays. Each week, we planned activities such as camping trips and friendly competitions to see who could roast or bake the best cake. These moments were filled with laughter, fun, and camaraderie, making the summer memorable.

As time moved on, our troop began preparing for the fall. With the new school year approaching, we geared up for our annual Girl Scout cookie sales. The excitement of organizing activities and looking forward to cookie season helped make the transition from summer into the school year smooth and enjoyable.

Unlike my initial experience in first grade, the start of the new school year soon became familiar. Every morning, my friends and I met at the same corner, walking to school together and sharing stories about our summer adventures. We grew comfortable with our daily schedule, knowing exactly when lunchtime was and when the bell would ring for dismissal.

As I settled into my routine, I made sure to complete my homework each day. After school, I often joined my friends to jump rope and play new games we learned. Weekends brought added excitement with our Girl Scout meetings, which gave us a sense of community and something to look forward to.

One morning before school, Dad told me that David Lee was going into the Army. While I was getting ready, David Lee explained that he would be leaving for a while. At that age, I didn't understand what the Army was, so I asked if I could go with him. He smiled and said, "No, you have school." We hugged, and he promised he would return soon.

David Lee said he was happy I had friends now and reminded me that I would be busy, especially with the holidays coming up. When Dad mentioned my friends were waiting outside, I joined them with tears still in my eyes. When they asked why I was crying, I told them David Lee was leaving for the Army. One of my friends mentioned her brother returned from the Army with a wife. We laughed about how someone could find a wife in the Army. Sharing jokes helped make the moment easier.

A few weeks later, I came home from school and found Dad there—unusual, since he was normally at work. He looked upset and unsure what to do. I sat on his lap to comfort him. Soon, people began arriving at our house, which was also unusual. Shirley Jean called me over and told me that Grandma Mae, my father's mother, had gone to heaven.

I asked Shirley Jean, "Why does everyone go to heaven?"

She said that when I grow older, I would understand. When I asked at what age, she told me to ask Bea, who would explain when the time was right.

Bea was home, and my older sister Katie had arrived; I usually only saw her at church. My Aunt Janie was there, along with my Aunt Kutchie and her husband, Uncle Cleo, who was close to Dad. My father—usually known for his outgoing personality—was different that day. Seeing him cry was unfamiliar and affected me deeply. I began to cry too, knowing I would no longer be visiting the country.

Uncle Cleo shared stories about Grandma Mae—her strength, her pride, and her Native identity. She never changed her style to please anyone. Though people sometimes called her unkind names, she was unaffected. My dad and brothers, however, never tolerated anyone disrespecting her. The townspeople learned quickly not to cross them.

Dad's demeanor changed after her passing. Family members said it would take time, especially since he had been an only child after his younger sister died at around five years old. He hadn't seen his biological father in years, but his bond with his mother was especially strong.

Grandma Mae and my father often communicated through expressions and codes only they understood. During visits to her home, my sister Kathy joined in activities, and I often played along with code words because Grandma Mae knew I loved them.

Grandma and Aunt Bobby Jean communicated in Pig Latin whenever Bea wasn't around. Grandma knew several coded languages.

She was known for her distinctive style—colorful moccasins, buckskin dresses, and braided hair decorated beautifully. Everything she wore matched perfectly. She carried herself with wisdom, strength, and pride. Both Dad and I felt her absence deeply. He knew how much I loved visiting her in the country.

Between the ages of eight and nine, I had moments that shaped my understanding of family. One day, Aunt Barbara Jean came to our house carrying a bottle in her purse. I watched as she secretly drank from that bottle. Even at that age, I noticed that the more she drank, the louder she became.

I was sitting behind the door as usual. She saw me and called out, telling me to come out, but I didn't move. She brought up Grandma Mae going to heaven. I simply said yes.

She began using coded words, asking if I knew what they meant. My brothers laughed. Then she made a harsh comment about Grandma Mae—calling her crazy and saying she once hit Dad in the ear with a shovel, which was why he couldn't hear well. The story made me cry.

One brother threatened to tell Dad I was crying. Shirley Jean overheard and asked what happened. The boys explained that Aunt Barbara Jean told me the story. Aunt Barbara insisted it was true and said someone needed to tell me that Grandma Mae wasn't a nice person. Shirley Jean told her she needed to leave before Bea or Dad came home. Aunt Barbara refused at first but eventually left with the boys.

Confused, I asked Shirley Jean why Grandma Mae would hit Dad with a shovel. Shirley Jean said she didn't know—Dad never said that. She wondered if maybe one of Grandma's husbands had done it, but she wasn't sure.

I also told her I noticed Aunt Barbara jean drank from a bottle in her purse while Dad drank from a bottle in his back pocket. To me, they seemed to be drinking the same thing—just in different ways.

As I grew more aware of whiskey and its effects, I also noticed Bea's frustration. Their arguments became more frequent and tense because of Dad's drinking.

One afternoon after school, I was at a friend's house when someone pointed out Dad walking toward us. Worried he came to find me, I ran to him. He seemed unlike himself, the bottle sticking from his pocket. Embarrassed, I loudly told my friends I would be back later. When I asked Dad to go home, he refused—until I began to cry.

Once home, I told Shirley Jean Dad had been drinking. She told him he shouldn't drink alcohol. When I said "whiskey," she explained whiskey *is* alcohol and that it makes people drunk. When I asked what "drunk" meant, she told me to look at Dad— his behavior was the answer.

Seeing my brothers in the house, I left to join my friends.

The next day, David Lee returned from the Army. He laughed and said he looked behind the door for me, expecting me to be in my usual spot. The family joked about how often I hid there—that it had become my signature place.

While he was away, we wrote letters and made phone calls to stay connected. These exchanges gave him support and kept our bond strong.

As Dad's alcohol use increased, our household grew tense. The sense of comfort faded, replaced by uncertainty. Bea noticed the changes quickly and grew more frustrated as interactions between her and Dad became louder and more frequent.

After his Army service, David Lee got his own place nearby, like most of our family. He stayed connected to us.

My sister Missie met one of David Lee's friends, who had returned from the Army. While David Lee stayed home, Missie's boyfriend transferred to the Air Force. She looked for a letter every day. Missie didn't spend much time at home and often stayed with friends.

She and my brother George had a close bond. They talked mostly to each other and kept to themselves. They avoided my teenage brothers—who we all called "Bea's boys"—and stayed out of Bea's way too.

When Missie's boyfriend returned home for a visit, the house felt excited. I overheard him telling Bea he wanted to marry Missie. Bea listened and agreed to his proposal. It was a significant moment for our family.

The next morning, I shared the news with my friends at school. I also mentioned that Dad didn't seem to like Missie's fiancé. Since Dad usually liked everyone, this surprised them.

When they asked if I had seen him face-to-face, I explained that I had only heard his voice during visits. This left me with unanswered questions.

Bea welcomed him warmly when he visited, treating him like family immediately. Dad, however, was quietly disapproving. He didn't argue, but his silence spoke loudly.

I felt confused, standing behind the door like always, watching and listening.

Changes in Dad's behavior grew more noticeable. He came home more often and drank more, despite Bea's clear dislike of alcohol in the house. The atmosphere shifted—subtle at first, then undeniable.

Bea made the rules, and Dad usually respected them. Anyone who didn't had to leave. That's how it had always been. But now, Dad was challenging those rules.

One morning before school, I noticed Dad asleep in the chair with an unfamiliar, almost angry expression. I lied to my friends, saying I couldn't play after school. I knew Missie's fiancé would be coming over, and I wanted to hide in my favorite place behind the door to understand why Dad disliked him.

I had never heard Dad raise his voice the way Bea did. Being near him used to make me feel safe. Now, I felt unsure.

That afternoon, when there was a knock on the door, I stayed hidden while my sister answered. She was excited to see him. From behind the door, I heard him ask who I was and why I was always hiding. My sister said I was just very shy.

The next morning, my friends immediately asked if I had seen Missie's fiancé. We joked about how my friend's brother came home with a wife, and David Lee came home with a brother-in-law.

I told them Dad didn't like him, which surprised them again.

Later, when I finally saw Missie's fiancé myself, David Lee called out to me, trying to bring me out from behind the door. I stayed hidden. Bea was home, and for once, I felt safer because of it.

I told my friends I had seen him and that he seemed nice. We tried to figure out why Dad was bothered when no one else was. I told them Dad had been drinking from a bottle. One friend said some men drink from bottles and women from glasses. I joked that my Aunt Barbara Jean drank from bottles like the men do. We laughed together.

Chapter 8:
Eyes of the Unknown

At ten years old, I began to notice something peculiar—
something I had sensed as early as age four. Whenever the town's
older ladies spoke to Bea in my presence, their behavior changed.
Even though I stood right beside her, they spoke *around* me, as if I
were invisible. Their voices carried the same uneasy instruction
every time:

"Tell her don't look at me."

The way they said it made it seem as though I possessed some
kind of strange power I couldn't understand. Their repeated
warnings left me confused and unsettled. Eventually, I turned to
Bea, hoping she could explain why they reacted this way. Her
response was calm, almost dismissive. She told me not to pay them
any mind. But her reassurances did little to quiet the questions still
swirling in my mind.

My curiosity only grew. I wanted to know why they focused on
my eyes, why they seemed so wary of me. When I asked again, Bea
finally said the women were afraid of "the gift" I had. But she never
explained what that gift was. Instead, her words only raised more
questions.

Seeking Answers About My Gift

One day, I asked, "If it's really a gift, why are the ladies afraid of me?" The question had been weighing on my mind for some time. Their unease and the way they avoided looking directly at me made me wonder what it was about me that unsettled them so much. Despite Bea's attempts to reassure me, I couldn't shake my curiosity or the feeling of being different from everyone else.

Bea answered with unusual patience. She said I needed to stay close to God and be grateful for the guidance I was given. When I asked what would happen if I didn't listen, she warned, "You'll regret it."

Feeling overwhelmed, I asked her, "You had twelve children— why am I the one?"

Her reply was firm:

"Never question God."

Her calm tone was something I hadn't heard before. It made her words feel even heavier.

When I asked how the ladies even knew who I was—since I never spoke to them—Bea said they reacted out of fear because they didn't know me. My presence was unfamiliar, and people fear what they do not understand. That uncertainty alone was enough to unsettle them.

Bea changed the subject, reminding me that my sister's wedding was the next day. The ceremony would be held at the pastor's home, and she said we had much to prepare. I didn't understand the significance of this, but Bea was focused on making sure everything went smoothly.

Soon after, Bea received an invitation to visit my sister and her husband at his mother's home, who lived in another part of town. It was unusual for Bea to accept such invitations—she always said,

"Sudden visits make long friendships." Usually, it was my sister Kathy who accompanied her, not me. when Bea told me I had to go along, I was confused and uneasy, especially knowing how the older women reacted around me.

When we arrived, Bea rang the doorbell. An excited lady answered and invited us in. She asked Bea who she had brought with her, and Bea said, "This is my baby." From her tone alone, I could tell she had a purpose for bringing me.

My sister and her husband were sitting on the sofa. Her husband smiled and said, "You're a cute little girl—stop hiding behind that door." Bea quickly told him I had always favored that spot.

Then his mother looked directly at me and asked, **"Where did she get those eyes from?"**

I froze. Once again, an older woman seemed bothered by my eyes. I lowered my head and quietly whispered to Bea that I wanted to go home. His mother added, "Tell her not to put those eyes on me," and the discomfort in the room was unmistakable. I held tightly to Bea's arm until she understood I couldn't stay another moment.

On the way home, I asked her again why these women were afraid of my eyes. Bea repeated what she always said:

"Remember, I told you God gifted some people... and you are one of them."

That night, I couldn't sleep. Their words and the dread in their voices replayed in my mind. Something about their fear felt dark— nothing like the warm mothers at my friends' homes. Those older women carried an energy I couldn't explain, and it frightened me. I didn't want to be near them. I didn't want them near me.

I lay awake for nights, trying to understand why they saw something in me that I couldn't see myself. The confusion became so heavy that I withdrew from everyone—including Bea. Her words only added to the uncertainty I felt.

I was terrified my friends would find out. I believed that if they knew what the older women said about me, they would never want to play with me again. The fear of losing them made me guard this secret closely.

One afternoon while shopping, I found myself staring at mirrors. The thought of buying one tugged at me, though I couldn't explain why. Bea noticed and asked why I wanted a mirror. I didn't know how to answer. She simply said, "There's one in the house," and walked on.

Throughout my childhood, I cherished a secret sanctuary—a quiet place that belonged only to me. Even at ten, I sought refuge there. It was the only place I felt truly safe, away from the chaos and the things I didn't understand. It was where I could think, breathe, and hide when the world felt too heavy.

One day, while I sat in front of a mirror at home, Bea said something that stayed with me:

"You can look in that mirror all day and not know what to look for.

If you pray, God will reveal it.

You don't have to search for what God has for you—remember that."

Her words unsettled me. Bea always seemed to know what I was thinking before I said it. Somehow, she was always one step ahead. It frightened me—and comforted me at the same time.

Chapter 9:
Loss, Family, and Endurance

The morning was perfect—neither too cold nor too hot—reminding us that winter was coming to an end and spring was just around the corner. For us Southerners, the month of March is something we look forward to each year. It brings a comfortable in-between season, where the harshness of winter fades and the warmth of spring begins to take hold. The air carries a sense of optimism and renewal, making it a favorite time for many in the South.

As my sister Katie's family and my aunt Janie's family grew, they relocated to larger homes to fit their expanding households. Even with these changes, our family always lived close to one another. There was never a reason for distance—Madea had raised her children and grandchildren to care for each other, and Bea continued the same tradition. My older siblings grew up closely bonded, always ready to stand up for one another. Supporting family was a value deeply rooted in our elders and carried down through generations.

Madea also made sure no one ever went hungry. Her pantry was always stocked, and behind her house she tended a flourishing garden filled with fresh vegetables and greens. A chicken coop in the backyard provided eggs and poultry year-round. Because of

Madea's dedication and resourcefulness, food was never a worry. Bea's prayers always ended with gratitude. After expressing thanks, she finished every prayer by thanking God—and she encouraged me to do the same, keeping our family grounded in faith and appreciation.

Shirley Jean eventually began caring for her own family, after years of raising Bea's children. She had started helping Bea when she was only nine years old, gaining the skills needed to manage a household long before she had her own. That early experience shaped her deeply, influencing the strong, capable woman she became.

When my sister Katie moved, Shirley Jean relocated to the house right n. This close proximity reflected the family tradition of staying near one another. It made it easier to help one another, stay connected, and support each other through the challenges of everyday life.

One afternoon, as my friends and I walked home from school, we heard sirens. People were running in the same direction we were headed. Even though the weather was cold, we barely noticed as we talked about our day, enjoying the routine we shared every afternoon. My house was the first stop on our walk home. As we approached, we saw smoke rising in the distance.

We immediately ran toward it—the smoke was coming from the same direction as my home. The closer we got, the clearer it became that something was terribly wrong. Neighbors and family members were running ahead, drawn by alarm and fear. The chill in the air disappeared as panic took over. By the time we reached the area, the scene was chaotic: a fire truck, an ambulance, and a large crowd stood outside.

It was my sister Shirley Jean's house—right next door to ours.

My family was outside, distressed and frantic. I saw an ambulance pulling away. I left my friends and ran toward my family.

In the chaos, everyone was desperately searching for my niece, Dwanna, who they believed was still inside the burning house. They checked her favorite spot—the clothes basket in the bedroom, where she often curled up and fell asleep among the warm, freshly washed laundry. It was a peaceful place she loved.

When they found the clothes basket, the reaction was immediate and devastating. Dwanna was there, lying as if she were sleeping—but the truth quickly became clear. She had passed away from smoke inhalation. The loss was crushing, leaving a deep wound in our entire family.

I asked Bea why she was covered and what had happened to Shirley Jean's baby. Bea softly replied, "She went to be with God." I was confused and heartbroken. "Why did He take her baby? Everyone says she died from smoke inhalation," I said through tears.

As Bea walked with our family down the street, I continued asking questions about those who had passed away. I remembered when Madea went to heaven to be with Granddaddy, and when Grandma Mae passed and went to heaven too. I wanted to know where God had taken Shirley Jean's child. Bea simply said, "Heaven."

This was an experience I would never forget. Bea reminded me that I had attended Sunday school and church all my life, and that everything we learned related back to God. She said, "One day *you* will die too. Everyone will. It's universal." Her words frightened me. When we arrived at my sister's house that night, I was scared to sleep. I worried I might die too. I cried uncontrollably, overwhelmed by grief and fear. Part of me thought that if I had known this would happen, I never would have come here.

Bea told me I had no choice. I disagreed silently—Bea had eleven children before me. Feeling powerless only made everything hurt more.

Bea then explained that my sister would be gone for a long time. She told me that my sister had suffered burns over ninety percent of her body. The severity meant her recovery would be long and uncertain. The weight of that reality settled over all of us.

I felt heartbroken knowing there would be a funeral for the baby—and my sister would be unable to attend. Bea told me my sister didn't know her baby had died and that we could not tell her because she was in too much pain. My heart ached for both of them. Bea took care of Shirley Jean's older daughter during this time.

The fire devastated our family, destroying everything we owned. Precious belongings—my toys, my coloring books, Sam, and countless keepsakes—were all gone. Every memory tied to those items was reduced to ashes. Our sense of security vanished with them.

After the fire, my siblings were forced to separate, each staying with different households across the area. The separation added another layer of trauma, making it harder to find comfort during such a painful time. Being split apart from one another when we needed each other most made the tragedy even heavier.

As Bea and Dad searched for a new place for us to live, each of us had to adjust to unfamiliar environments. The transition was difficult. We were all coping with trauma in different ways, and being apart only intensified the loneliness and fear.

Still, in times of difficulty, our family's closeness showed. Whenever something happened, everyone gathered—never more than a block or two away. This closeness ensured that even in crisis, no one was ever truly alone.

Months later, my sister finally returned home from the hospital. Though she survived, she was physically weak and emotionally fragile. Her recovery was long and painful. But despite everything, she never lost her faith in God. She talked to Him every day— sometimes all day. The more she cried out to Him, the stronger she seemed to become. Her trust in God remained unshaken, even though He now held her baby in His care. Family and friends gathered around her often, offering comfort and support. After some time, she found a house and moved in with her older daughter.

As I grew older, I became more aware of my surroundings. I stayed active in the community and spent a lot of time with my friends. Bea didn't like this shift at all. I didn't know what was going on between Bea and Dad, and I didn't want to know. I just stayed busy.

I began learning things about myself—especially how I felt around my family. No sibling was going to tell *me* what to do—I refused to accept it. Bea noticed that I wasn't listening to her or anyone else. I said their too many bosses" around me. Now she wanted to control me as if I were still a little girl.

I told Bea I deserved to act my age. She didn't like my mouth, my new friends, or my independence. She wanted full control over me. But I wasn't afraid anymore. The beatings and punishments didn't affect me—I had grown numb to the pain. I spoke my mind freely. Bea thought I was crazy because I would fight my brothers or anyone who put their hands on me. I told her she needed to talk to her kids about putting their hands on me. I wasn't having it.

My anger toward Dad's constant absence and unpredictable presence continued to grow. His coming and going left a void I didn't know how to fill. I found myself lashing out more whenever

Bea criticized me or tried to control me. Her voice felt overwhelming, and I grew tired of her always trying to manage every part of my life.

After Dad moved more accurately, after Bea made the decision for him to leave—he found a place to live on the other side of town. I would visit him often, sometimes feeling sad about the circumstances. Despite the distance and the separation, there was a noticeable absence of the usual arguments and noise between Dad and Bea. However, Bea's need for control persisted. She continued to exert influence over Dad, either by stopping by his workplace herself or by sending one of us check on him.

Even after Dad and Bea physically separated, Bea's need to maintain influence over Dad's life never seemed to waver. One day, while stopping by Dad's house, I was surprised to find another woman in the kitchen, cooking as if she belonged there. Dad greeted me with a smile and introduced her as his friend. She moved comfortably around the kitchen, clearly familiar with the space, and spoke to me as though she had known me for years, even calling me "Dad's baby."

As I stood there, I immediately thought about Bea. I knew I wasn't going to say a word to her about Dad's new companion. If she found out, she would likely come over to the house, and the ensuing commotion would make its way around town. I didn't want to face the embarrassment of their actions being the latest subject of gossip. The situation left me feeling caught in the middle, trying to protect my own sense of peace amid the ongoing family drama.

As I began to visit Dad more frequently at his new home, I found myself pleasantly surprised by the atmosphere that awaited me there. The woman he had introduced as his friend proved to be quite pleasant and welcoming. The house, which had once been filled with the noise and tension of family arguments when Bea stops over, now felt peaceful and calm in her presence.

She greeted me warmly and tried to make me feel comfortable, often engaging me in friendly conversation. Over time, I grew to appreciate her kindness and the genuine care she showed. Dad had told her that my favorite pie was blueberry, and she took it upon herself to bake it for me often. This simple gesture made me feel seen and valued, bringing a small comfort amid the ongoing changes in our family. Her thoughtfulness and the quiet she brought to the house helped create a space where I could relax and enjoy my visits with Dad.

The boys' decision to report on my visits to Bea only fueled the conflict, cutting off my contact with Dad and deepening the rift. Now, with Dad moving so far away, Bea's influence over him diminished, she could no longer control his life as she once did. Yet, her insistence on receiving what she called "her money" kept a thread of connection alive, one that Dad felt obligated to maintain to avoid further trouble. The distance provided some relief, but the underlying disputes and demands continued to shape our family's interactions, leaving me longing for peace I desperately needed. The constant push and pull of expectations and loyalties made it harder to find my own space within the chaos, intensifying my desire to be respected and left alone.

With Dad gone, my brothers started trying to discipline me, acting as if they were now in charge. Their attempts to assert authority did nothing but increase the tension within our family, and I immediately felt the negative impact. I didn't want any part of their interference—especially when it came to my choice of friends. They felt entitled to tell me who I could spend time with, but I refused to accept that kind of control. The situation only became more complicated, and their involvement pushed me even further away, strengthening my resolve to make my own decisions without their influence.

Sometimes, I wondered if there was something about me that I didn't understand—something the women in town knew and never explained. The thought made me feel even more out of place.

More than anything, I wanted space and autonomy. I wanted to be left alone in the places where I felt most comfortable. I wanted control over my own feelings and decisions. I wanted others to respect my need for independence.

What made the situation even more difficult was my brother's insistence on disciplining me, as though he had the authority to dictate my actions. His attempts to assert control only fueled my resentment and highlighted his overstepping role in the family.

Rather than feeling supported, I felt increasingly isolated, with his interference making it even harder to find peace or belonging within the household.

At times, I questioned whether there was something about myself that I was missing—some secret understanding that the women in town possessed but had never shared with me. This uncertainty deepened my sense of alienation, making me feel even more out of place in my own environment.

Above all, I craved space and autonomy. I longed for the freedom to be left alone in the places where I felt most at ease, to have control over my emotions and the choices I made. More than anything, I wanted others to acknowledge and respect my need for independence, allowing me the dignity to make my own decisions without interference.

Chapter 10:
Discovering Who I am

During my teenage years between fourteen and fifteen, I frequently found myself surrounded by family members who did not hesitate to express their opinions about the friends I chose and the decisions I made. Their voices were often the loudest in the room, and their judgments felt constant and unrelenting. Despite my efforts to assert my own views or defend my preferences, it seemed as if my thoughts carried little weight within the family dynamic. This persistent disregard left me feeling invisible and unheard, struggling to carve out a space where my voice mattered. Over time, the repeated dismissal of my feelings and choices only deepened my sense of isolation and frustration, making it clear just how challenging it was to be understood in my own home.

As a result, I frequently chose to withdraw from these exchanges rather than actively participate. This became a coping mechanism, helping me avoid the tension and discomfort that came with conflicting viewpoints. By stepping back, I hoped to find some peace, even if it meant my feelings and ideas went unheard.

Bea seemed troubled by the way I communicated, especially when I tried to stand up for my own needs. Whenever I tried to advocate for myself, her response was often marked by concern and, at times, outright resistance.

I often found myself emotionally and physically drained after interacting with Bea's children. Each encounter seemed to sap my energy, leaving me feeling depleted and frustrated. Despite my repeated requests for Bea to step in and ask her children not to reprimand me, my frustrations only intensified over time. The lack of intervention made these exchanges even more difficult to endure, as my appeals for understanding were frequently overlooked.

While I did my best to respect Bea's approach to parenting and acknowledge her authority within the family, I found it challenging to extend that same respect to her children when it came to disciplinary matters. Their involvement felt inappropriate and unwelcome, heightening my sense of discomfort and isolation within the household. As a result, I was left struggling to cope with the ongoing tensions, wishing for boundaries that would allow me the space and autonomy I needed.

Bea openly shared with others that I was to blame for the challenges within our family, which only intensified my feelings of alienation. Being singled out in this way made me feel even more isolated and misunderstood. The physical punishments I endured were already overwhelming, and while I acknowledged that discipline was a common practice in Bea's family, I found it deeply unpleasant and difficult to accept. The combination of being blamed for family problems and subjected to harsh discipline left me struggling to cope with my circumstances, reinforcing my desire for acceptance and understanding.

One statement I can make with confidence is that Bea never committed an ass whipping without following through. I didn't complain, but I told Bea that her children shouldn't touch me because I was already uncomfortable when she did. I made it clear that if this ever happened, I would take appropriate action to protect myself.

Larry, my youngest brother, was known for his strong temperament. He had reached a point in his life where my actions no longer affected or concerned him, marking a shift in our relationship compared to earlier years. Our bond had been shaped, in part, by shared experiences—like the incident with our sister and the knife. These moments influenced how we related to each other and how we navigated the complexities of our family environment.

Despite the challenges within our household, Larry often appeared unaware or disconnected when Bea placed her hand on either me or him. His demeanor suggested a certain detachment from the disciplinary actions that occurred. Notably, Larry no longer endured physical discipline at his age, which set him apart from some of the experiences I faced. This distinction further highlighted the evolving roles and boundaries among siblings as we grew older.

One might expect that my brother Frank would experience some guilt regarding the incident that occurred during my childhood, and that Bea might recognize her lack of intervention in protecting me. Here we go—he put his hands on me, and Bea did nothing. He pushed me to the floor several times, and I kept getting up; like I said, I would fight until death if anyone put their hands on me.

Frank wanted to control me—why, I don't know. I had not forgotten what happened to the little girl behind that door. He had issues with me, and even my sister—whom I once thought was mentally challenged—was now pulling a knife on me. Bea allowed her boys to discipline me, and that did not go well with me. I told Bea, "God said: honor thy mother and father, that thy days shall be long." That is the fifth commandment. I will honor that.

The ongoing attempts to control me remained a source of confusion and frustration. Despite not understanding the reasons behind this need for dominance, I still carried the memory of what happened to the little girl behind that door. She lived within me, and I was determined to protect her for the rest of my life.

Bea maintained close relationships with the sheriff, judges, Indian chiefs and other influential white officials in town. Her reputation among these individuals was well established, and she often gave significant priority to their opinions and directives. Whenever challenges or conflicts arose within our household, Bea did not hesitate to confide in these authorities and seek their guidance on how to proceed.

Whenever family issues arose, Bea consistently chose to share her own viewpoint with external parties and followed the guidance provided by those authorities. Her approach often involved consulting with individuals in positions of power, such as sheriffs, judges, and other influential community members. I questioned Bea's emphasis on knowing these officials, expressing my confusion about why such connections were necessary in our personal lives. To this, Bea responded that, in her view, having connections with people of influence was essential. She believed that without these relationships, one could easily find themselves facing serious trouble, saying, "If you're in this world and don't have connections, you will find yourself in jail or hell."

Recently, Bea reached out to the authorities regarding the challenges she was experiencing with me. However, the account she provided was entirely from her perspective, representing only her own interpretation of events. This reliance on external officials and her tendency to prioritize their opinions significantly affected how issues were addressed within our household. Bea's approach not only shaped decisions but influenced the overall dynamics of our family—often leaving me feeling unheard and misunderstood.

One evening, I decided to spend time at the local club with my friends, a familiar gathering spot for teenagers in our community. The atmosphere was typical—filled with laughter, music, and conversation. As I enjoyed my time, my brother Frank arrived and spotted me inside.

Frank's reaction was immediate and disruptive. In front of my friends and everyone present, he loudly instructed me to leave the club. His intervention was both embarrassing and confusing, especially since Frank had no authority over me. His decision to assert control over me only underscored the tense power dynamics within our family.

When I arrived home that evening, I discovered that Frank had beaten me there. He immediately began speaking with Bea, sharing false accounts about my behavior at the club. Frank was determined to portray me negatively, twisting the events to suit his own narrative.

As he continued to tell his version of the story, I confronted him directly. I firmly told Frank that he had no right or authority over me, making it clear that his attempts to control or discipline me were unacceptable. The exchange underscored the power struggles and misunderstandings that often arose within our family, especially when the truth became distorted by personal agendas.

After the confrontation with Frank, I tried to explain to Bea what had happened. Frank pushed me to the floor, and each time I managed to get up, he pushed me down again. Despite the repeated aggression, I refused to give up, and Bea witnessed my persistence firsthand. On the final push, I landed with my ear caught on the pointed end of the coffee table. Blood began dripping from the injury, but I continued to stand my ground.

Once Frank went outside, I quickly went to the phone and called my brother David Lee, who lived nearby. I asked him to take me to the hospital so I could receive medical attention.

David Lee arrived, and Frank had made it back inside the house. I will say this—Frank got a can of whoopa.

David Lee and I tried to stop the bleeding. He said we were going to the hospital because it looked like it needed stitches. Before leaving, as I walked to David Lee's car, I screamed, telling Bea what I was going to do to her son when I got back.

We arrived at the hospital; the blood continued to flow. I was seen immediately, and the wound required stitches. After we left, it was late. David Lee said I didn't need to go back to the house—that Bea and Frank needed time to calm down.

After the incident, I spent the night with David Lee and his family. It was familiar; no matter what happened, I always ended up at David Lee's house, sometimes for long periods.

Whenever I stayed longer than expected, Bea would eventually call him and request—just as she always did—that he bring me back home. The repetition never made sense to me. Each time David Lee prepared to take me back, I tried to explain my reluctance.

I told him plainly that I did not want to return. My fear was real and persistent. I knew that if I went back, someone was going to get hurt—and I was certain it wouldn't be me.

Throughout these experiences, I noticed a pattern in the way my siblings, especially David Lee and Katie, interacted with Bea. Neither of them ever confronted her or pointed out when she was in the wrong. Instead, it seemed as though they held Bea to a standard that they were unwilling to question or challenge. Their silence reinforced the unspoken boundaries within our family, where certain behaviors went unchecked and authority was rarely contested. This dynamic contributed to the ongoing misunderstandings and left me feeling isolated whenever I tried to address issues directly.

During this period, I made it clear that I would not tolerate being beaten or mistreated by anyone. My resolve was firm. No matter what challenges arose, I would not accept being hurt by anyone.

Bea's friends expressed concern and suggested that I see a counselor. Acting on their advice, Bea arranged for counseling sessions. My brother David Lee informed me that I now had appointments scheduled three times a week after school. The sudden need for these frequent visits left me confused, questioning the decision, as I felt nothing was wrong with me.

In our family of twelve children, I was the first to be sent to counseling. Bea often attributed this to my outspoken nature, claiming that my "mouth" being direct straightforward in communication.

She handed me an address and clearly stated the time I was expected to be there.

I was always with my friends after school—now I had to report to this office. My friends asked where I was going. "I must see a counselor three times a week," I said. Of course, they wanted to know why. "Bea said it's my mouth." My friend said, "You're just like her—wow. My dad said the same about me."

I walked to the building and told the lady I had an appointment. She advised me to take a seat. Minutes later, she said the counselor would see me and led me into his office. A white man in a suit—not looking like a doctor to me—said, "Come in and have a seat."

I was afraid.

He began by asking what brought me there and what had been happening. Throughout the session, he asked questions and drew sketches on paper. This made the interaction feel less formal and helped me open up. The drawings seemed to reflect what he heard, and I found myself responding more comfortably.

The session lasted about an hour. I began to enjoy it... someone actually heard me. I started looking forward to our visits; he always had my favorite snacks. After weeks of visiting, the more open I became—about Bea, Dad, my siblings, and my friends. I was able to escape the noise and discover who I was. It became one of the most profound moments of my life.I possessed a strong sense of self, which may explain why some older women in town had concerns about me. As Bea often said, I seemed to have

Each night, as I lay down to sleep, I found comfort in watching the stars. Their gentle glow seemed to make my dreams more vivid, and in those dreams, I was often rescued by someone I couldn't quite identify—always white men in white coats. I never fully understood why this image appeared so often, but perhaps it was because, in those moments, I longed for protection and safety that I rarely felt during the day.

The solace I discovered in these nighttime reveries became my own private escape. It was a quiet space where the confusion and tension of my daily life faded away, and where hope quietly began to take root. As I reflected on the counselor's words, they echoed in my mind, urging me to look beyond Mississippi and trust that I was meant for something different, something greater than what my family could offer.

With every step forward, I carried the memory of starlit nights and the belief that I could shape my own future, no matter how uncertain the path ahead might be. The quiet comfort I found in watching the stars each night stayed with me, reminding me that hope could exist even in the most challenging circumstances. Despite the confusion and tension that filled my days, those moments under the night sky gave me strength and reassurance. They became a source of inspiration, helping me trust in my own resilience and guiding me as I moved toward independence. The dreams I had under those stars fed my determination to seek something greater for myself and to believe that I could build a better life beyond the world I knew.

The counselor told me, after all these visits and getting to know me: "You don't need to come back. This is your last visit." He said I was well-knowledgeable for my age—far above my years. He told me that I had outgrown my family due to the experiences and challenges I had faced.

"The best advice I can give you," he said, "is to leave the state of Mississippi when you get old enough. I'm sure you don't belong here and will do much better when you leave." He handed me an envelope and said, "Give this to your mother. Tell her you will be fine, and if she has questions, she can call me."

I left feeling good.

I knew I didn't fit in. I was right all along—I was different from my family. The gift was right.

Final Visit.

Chapter 11:
The Path to Independence

During the summer when I was fifteen, I found myself eagerly anticipating the arrival of fall and my sixteenth birthday. The thought of turning sixteen filled me with excitement and a sense of possibility. More than anything, I wanted to visit my dad in Chicago. The idea of spending time with him and experiencing a change of scenery was something I looked forward to with hope. However, when I asked Bea for permission to make the trip, she refused. Her answer was a simple and firm "no," leaving me disappointed and frustrated as I continued to dream about the visit that would not happen.

After spending time with my friends and assuming I would be home for the summer, everything suddenly changed one afternoon. When I returned from my friend's house, Bea told me that my sister Missie had called from Oklahoma. Missie was living on a military base in Altus, Oklahoma, and she wanted to know if I could come and babysit her son and daughter for the summer.

To my surprise and excitement, Bea agreed and gave permission for me to go. As soon as I received the news, I immediately called my friend to share what had happened and to let them know I would be traveling to visit my sister. The prospect of spending the summer with Missie in Oklahoma filled me with anticipation, and I looked forward to the new experiences awaiting me on the base.

It was an incredible experience, and I truly enjoyed my time there. My sister even asked Bea if I could stay and attend school, but Bea refused and insisted that I return home. The journey back to Mississippi was difficult and filled with frustration toward Bea. Throughout the trip, I couldn't shake the counselor's advice from my mind: *I needed to leave Mississippi.*

As the new school year approached, I told Bea that all my friends were attending a different school, and their bus ride was only about fifteen minutes. Bea said she would consider it. The very next morning, she agreed. I think she was simply worn out from saying no to me, especially after managing to bring me back home from Oklahoma.

Life settled a bit, and I spent more time with my friends, still thinking about how much I liked Altus, Oklahoma. Time passed quickly, and once again I asked Bea if I could visit Dad in Chicago—this time for Thanksgiving. Bea said, "You can go for Christmas." I called Dad to tell him I would be there for Christmas break.

I had fun. My dad's friend had two girls my age, and they kept me busy—shopping, riding buses across Chicago. I even visited my older brothers. I asked Bea if I could stay with Dad, and once again she said no, insisting that I needed to finish school back home.

After returning to Mississippi, I faced challenges at school that led to a major setback. I got into trouble, and the principal decided to suspend me for two weeks. This added tension at home, prompting Bea to reach out to Missie in Oklahoma to discuss the difficulties she was having with me.

During their conversation, Missie expressed her belief that a change of environment could be good for me. She suggested that if I returned to Oklahoma, it would give me a fresh start and the opportunity to meet new people.

To my surprise, Bea told me I would be going back to Oklahoma again. After all the times she had said no, I could hardly believe she was now saying yes. I went to stay with my sister and remained with her until the summer before my eighteenth birthday, when I left Oklahoma.

My friends from Mississippi moved to Chicago with the attention of getting a job and our own place. I asked Dad if I could come, and he said yes. Bea couldn't refuse—I would be grown in November, which meant I was going to be leaving soon either way.

All my friends returned to Chicago wanting to be "grown." Oh, what a price it costs to be grown—no more asking parents for help. When we did, we all heard the same answer: *You wanted to be grown, now take care of yourself and get a job.*

As we continued moving from house to house across Chicago, we began to realize that it was time to grow up. The freedom we imagined came with challenges. Dad frequently voiced his frustrations, complaining about Bea calling to say I needed to get a job. The pressure from our parents reminded us that independence came with responsibility.

We would look at one another and shrug. It was clear: if we wanted to be grown, we had to act grown. That meant finding work and taking care of ourselves, no longer relying on our parents.

During those days, my friends and I spent our time smoking weed, playing cards, and watching soap operas. We laughed together all day, making the most of whatever money we had. But eventually the money ran out. Smoking made us incredibly hungry, and the only food left was a pot of cold beans. I ended up eating the entire pot myself.

Afterward, I felt so bloated and uncomfortable that I couldn't move. Seeing my condition, my friend's sister decided it was best to tell them which hospital to take me to. The whole situation was sad and sobering.

It was deeply embarrassing when we arrived at the hospital. I explained to the doctor that I had smoked weed and eaten an entire pot of cold beans. The doctor told me to stand in the corner and touch my toes until he returned. Confused, I asked my friend why the doctor would have me do that—we thought it was absurd.

When the doctor returned, he explained I was suffering from flatulence. None of us understood what that meant. A nurse passed by, and one of my friends asked her. She explained—by bending over and touching her toes—that the doctor wanted the gas to release. And sure enough, just as predicted, once it started, my friends left even faster than the doctor.

This experience marked a turning point for me. The embarrassment and discomfort forced me to reflect on my choices and the consequences they carried.

Some of my friends eventually moved back home and got jobs. I went back to live with Dad. His friend had two daughters about one and two years older than me. They offered to give me a ride on Monday morning to apply for a job. When I arrived, the office told me I had to wait and come back in November when I turned eighteen. It was the end of September—I had almost two months to wait.

I asked if I could let my friend know I was leaving for the bus stop and that I had to wait until I turned eighteen. They told me the walk was long, and it was snowing. They asked if I wanted to wait in the break room until they got off work, but I said no. I needed to learn the bus route.

As I walked to the bus stop, the same guy my friends introduced me to came out of the building. Snow was falling hard, and the wind was blowing. He stopped to offer me a ride and said he remembered meeting me earlier. He asked if I got the job. I told him no—not yet. I explained I needed to be eighteen, and it was only the beginning of October. As I got out of the car, he asked my last name. I told him and said thanks for the ride.

I had no idea who was calling when the phone rang later that week. My aunt came into my room to tell me someone from the company was on the line. It was only Wednesday, and I had been there on Monday. Curious and anxious, I answered.

Let's just say—I got the job.

The first person I called was Bea. She was so proud and told me, "I knew you would do good." Her words meant everything in that moment.

As I entered adulthood, my relationship with Bea began to change. Now that I was working and supporting myself, I no longer needed to rely on Bea or Dad for financial help. This newfound independence brought me pride and a deep sense of accomplishment. For the first time, I could truly say I was grown— not just in age but in responsibility.

My friends in Mississippi would call and tell me how Bea bragged about me. How humble and proud she was of her baby.

Understanding a woman who didn't want to lose her child to the streets of Mississippi helped me make sense of her ways. Bea was fighting for something bigger than just me—her God and the battle she believed existed between us, tied to the gifts she claimed God had given.

Chapter 12:
Bea's Life Before and After Cancer

Bea's Strength and Sacrifice

Bea became a mother at just sixteen years old, and soon after, she welcomed more children into her life. The immense responsibility of raising a large family at such a young age was overwhelming. During those challenging years, Bea relied heavily on her parents, Madea and Granddaddy, for support. Their consistent involvement proved crucial, helping Bea manage the difficulties of young motherhood and ensuring her children were cared for while she worked toward building a stable future for her family.

When Bea needed to dedicate time to employment, Madea and Granddaddy took on the responsibility of caring for three of her children. Their willingness to step in allowed Bea to focus on building a future for herself and her family. With her parents' support, Bea secured a job working for a white family, where she helped raise their children while her own children were lovingly cared for by Madea and Granddaddy.

This arrangement gave Bea the opportunity to gain independence. Over time, her hard work enabled her to move into her own house, marking a significant milestone in her journey. Even after Bea established her own home, Madea continued to babysit her grandchildren so Bea could maintain her employment and provide for her family.

As Bea's family grew, Madea and Granddaddy's responsibilities increased. Bea had two additional children, and once again, her parents provided essential care so Bea could continue working. During this time, Bea's sister, Aunt Kutchie, also lived in the same house with her three children. This meant that Madea and Granddaddy were not only caring for Bea's children but also for the grandchildren from Aunt Kutchie, effectively managing a household with multiple young children.

Eventually, Bea married my dad and took all her children with her to begin a new chapter in their lives together. This transition marked an important shift for the entire family, as Bea's departure changed the caregiving responsibilities that had once been shared in the household.

After Bea moved out, Aunt Kutchie also entered a new phase of her life. She married and made the difficult decision to leave her three children in the care of Madea and Granddaddy. This choice reflected both her trust in her parents and the ongoing tradition of intergenerational support within the family.

Continuing the Cycle of Support

The pattern of family support continued with Bea's younger sister, Aunt Dorothy. When Aunt Dorothy returned home pregnant, she gave birth to a daughter and, like her sisters before her, left her child with Madea and Granddaddy. This ongoing cycle demonstrated the deep reliance on Madea and Granddaddy's care, as they once again opened their home and hearts to support their grandchildren and help their daughters pursue new paths.

Throughout these years, Madea and Granddaddy's unwavering dedication provided stability and support not only for Bea but for multiple generations within the family. Their home became a refuge and a foundation for their daughters and grandchildren, ensuring that everyone was cared for while the mothers worked to build better lives for their children.

During those times, the focus was simply on survival. Bea could not afford to live in fear; she had too many children who depended on her daily strength and perseverance. The burden of raising such a large family was immense, but Bea was fortunate to receive help from Shirley Jean. Even as a child, Shirley Jean played a crucial role in supporting her mother. At just nine years old, she managed the household, attended school, and completed her chores, helping to lighten Bea's load and keep the family running as smoothly as possible despite the many challenges they faced.

The unwavering determination and teamwork of Bea, Madea, Granddaddy, Shirley Jean, and the extended family served as a lifeline for us all, especially in our most difficult times. Bea became a better grandmother than a mother—I often heard it turns out like that. I just wanted to move out of the way of her and her grandchildren. Let's just say she turned into Madea.

Bea Continuing Madea's Legacy

Guidance within the family, providing care not only for her own children but also for her grandchildren. Bea was raised with numerous grandchildren who came in and out of her home. Her commitment to family echoed the unwavering dedication that Madea had shown, ensuring that the next generation received the same level of love, security, and structure that had been given to her.

This foundation of support was something I only began to truly appreciate as I matured into adulthood. It wasn't until I moved to Chicago that I fully understood the depth of Bea's struggles and the pain she carried—pain that had often gone unseen or unspoken when I was younger.

A Turning Point: Facing Bea's Diagnosis

Prior to Bea's diagnosis, Shirley Jean was on vacation visiting the family in Mississippi. Our oldest sister, Katie, recognized Shirley's reliability and asked her to take her son, Anthony, to a doctor's appointment located a few miles outside of town. Joining them on this trip was Shirley Jean's friend, Juanita, who offered additional company and support. This small act of helping with Anthony's appointment reflected the way family members leaned on each other during challenging times, relying on one another for both emotional and practical support.

After my nephew Anthony's appointment, my sister Katie and Juanita asked Shirley Jean if they could shop at a store in the area. Shirley Jean and my nephew chose to remain in the car while they shopped. After observing the area, they decided to walk across the highway instead of driving.

The traumatic accident occurred on August 27, 1978, leaving Shirley Jean with severe injuries that required her to be in a cast from her ankle all the way up to her hip. To make matters even more difficult, there was only one surgeon available in the area, and he had just recently suffered a heart attack, further complicating her treatment options.

During this challenging period, my cousin Malcolm played a crucial role in supporting the family. He flew from Milwaukee, Wisconsin, to Memphis, Tennessee, to pick up Shirley Jean and personally drove her back to Milwaukee in her own vehicle. Shirley Jean underwent numerous extensive surgeries to save her leg. Milwaukee is deeply connected to our family's history, a place where many generations before us raised their children and built lasting roots, even though she was miles away from the rest of us.

While Shirley Jean was undergoing these surgeries, Bea received her diagnosis of lung cancer. Despite her own recovery,

Shirley Jean made the difficult journey back to Mississippi with a full leg-to-thigh cast to care for her mother, demonstrating the unwavering commitment and strength that defined our family's approach to adversity.

Initially, I was not fully informed about Bea's illness. By the time I learned that Bea had been diagnosed with cancer, she was already getting ready for surgery to have one of her lungs removed. Even though I spoke to Bea on the phone every day—sometimes twice a day—she never mentioned her diagnosis directly, as if I already knew because we talked so frequently.

I noticed that every time I called Bea, she would get off the phone quickly, which was out of character for her. Bea had always loved to talk, and sharing knowledge was one of her specialties. This abrupt change in her behavior concerned me, so I mentioned to Dad that Bea seemed to have a cold.

When I expressed my growing concerns about Bea's health, Dad's reaction was immediate and intense. He shifted abruptly from his usual calm demeanor to agitation, insisting, "Bunion, you make everything big. You worry too much." Despite his attempt to downplay the situation and lighten the mood by reaching for a drink and joking that I was working on his nerves, my concern remained. I was determined to understand what was truly happening with Bea's health, especially since she repeatedly claimed to "just have a cold" every time we spoke.

Feeling unsettled by Bea's persistent claims and Dad's dismissiveness, I decided to contact my brother, David Lee, seeking clarity about Bea's condition. David Lee confirmed that Bea was indeed ill and explained that she had chosen not to tell me about her diagnosis immediately. She felt I was thriving in my job and living independently and did not want me to feel compelled to leave my work to be with her during this difficult time.

The moment I learned the truth about Bea's diagnosis marked a significant turning point for me. The steady path I had been following was suddenly disrupted, forcing me to face the harsh reality of her illness. This experience not only changed my outlook but also deepened my understanding of Bea and the immense challenges she had carried throughout her life.

Faced with the heartbreaking reality of Bea's illness, my dad and I realized we had to make a difficult, selfless decision. Together, we chose to leave Chicago and return home so that we could be there for Bea, offering her the support and care she needed during such a trying time. This was not an easy choice, but it was one made from love and a sense of family duty.

My sister Missie and her husband applied for a humanitarian assignment to be close to Bea as we all prepared to make the journey home to tend to her needs. They were eventually stationed at a location about three hours from Mississippi—the closest place available for his Air Force code. When Missie and her husband finally arrived, they stopped by Bea's house, where we gathered to update them on Bea's health and the situation at home. They explained their plans, saying they intended to visit Bea at the hospital before heading over to his family's home. With the house already overflowing with relatives and visitors, they invited me to stay with them in Arkansas, assuring me that I would have a place with them.

During this challenging period, my relatives emphasized the importance of family support, encouraging me to join them on their regular weekend trips to see Bea. Their invitation was more than just an offer to travel together—it represented a way for me to stay closely involved in Bea's care and to strengthen my connection with the rest of the family. These frequent visits provided a much-needed sense of belonging, allowing me to remain present and supportive despite the difficulties we were all facing. By participating in these gatherings, I was able to maintain meaningful ties with Bea and my loved ones, reinforcing the unity and resilience that defined our family during such trying times.

Even though the house looked just as I remembered—with the same furniture and familiar rooms—the experience of being there was overwhelming. Walking through each space, I was met with a flood of memories, each one carrying the weight of past struggles and the ongoing challenge of finding stability amid chaos. The home, never a place of comfort for me, now felt like a battleground where the fight for a sense of security and normalcy seemed never-ending.

Every room in the house was filled with my siblings and a steady stream of visiting relatives, their constant presence occupying every space and making it difficult to find any peace. The familiar of not quite belonging began to shift into a new discomfort restless, crowded energy that seemed to permeate every corner. The home, which I had long associated with trauma and a particular coldness, now felt strangely unfamiliar. The spaces I once knew were transformed, carrying an atmosphere that was both new and unsettling, sharply contrasting with my earlier memories. Instead of offering comfort, the house brought a sense of unease and disconnection, emphasizing how much—and yet how little—had truly changed during this difficult time.

Bea had one of her lungs removed, and we thought she would be okay after the surgery. My oldest sister, Katie, moved Bea into her home. Katie continued to work while her daughter, my niece Sheila, watched over Bea as family and friends visited throughout the day. I could see that Bea was weak and no longer the larger-than-life person I had known all my life. At times, there were simply too many visitors, and the constant company left her exhausted when she needed rest most.

Bea's Presence in the Community

Bea was widely respected in our community for her deep wisdom and thoughtful perspective, even though she seldom ventured out on her own. Whenever she encountered someone in town, she would gladly engage in long, meaningful conversations, offering insight and comfort to those around her.

As family members eagerly lined up, each waiting for their chance to visit Bea, I found myself consistently pushed to the end of the line, almost as if my presence were an afterthought. It became painfully obvious that my thoughts and feelings held little significance in those moments. No one really expected me to contribute, and even if I tried to speak up, I doubted my words would be heard or valued. At just twenty-one years old, most relatives seemed to assume I lacked the maturity or experience to grasp the seriousness of what was happening. Yet, deep down, I sensed that my understanding of the circumstances and their consequences was far greater than anyone gave me credit for— and perhaps even more profound than I realized myself.

When it was time for Bea to have a follow-up visit in Memphis, Tennessee, we discussed who would travel with her. It came down to "Bea's girls"—my oldest sister Katie, second-oldest Shirley Jean, third-oldest Missie, and myself, the youngest. Our sister Kathy stayed home; she had two children under the age of four.

Shirley Jean volunteered to drive. We weren't sure how she could manage it with a cast still on her leg, but she insisted. The trip to the doctor's office took about an hour and fifteen minutes. The visit itself seemed pleasant. He told us Bea was doing well. I didn't understand why she wasn't going to receive chemotherapy and was told she didn't need it. That explanation did not sit well with me.

On the way home, I saw a sign for Graceland and asked Bea if she wanted to ride by. She said yes. I knew she would be excited— she loved Elvis Presley and felt that only God could create a man so handsome. That slow drive-by put joy in her heart. I watched her shift and sit up in the car, taking it all in.

Not long after we returned home, we could see Bea wasn't getting better. It was all downhill from there. Bea was admitted back to the hospital, and the family was told she would not be coming home. Everyone prayed in their own way to the God they knew. Meanwhile, Bea was suffering.

Finally, Bea told my brother David Lee that she wanted to see me and asked him to bring me so I could spend the night. David Lee brought me the news: "She asked for her baby and wants to spend some time with you."

That night, I chose to stay over, allowing myself to be fully present with Bea. The time we spent together was incredibly meaningful to me. In the quiet and comfort of her presence, I felt immense joy and gratitude for the chance to share those private moments with her. Being alone with Bea gave us the space to connect deeply, uninterrupted by the usual stream of visitors and family. It remains one of the most cherished experiences of my life.

During one of our conversations, Bea explained why she had treated me differently than my sister Kathy, despite our closeness in age. She shared her observations of Kathy, noting that Kathy had always been needy due to her mental challenges. Kathy often whined and wandered off without a sense of judgment, making her more vulnerable in daily life.

Bea expressed her concern about Kathy's lack of discernment when it came to identifying safe situations or trustworthy people. This vulnerability, Bea explained, made Kathy more likely to leave the house with anyone, whether or not they were familiar or trustworthy. Bea's reflections highlighted her protective instincts and the unique considerations she faced in caring for Kathy compared to me.

Bea often remarked on the ways in which I reminded her of herself. She saw me as fearless—someone who was not easily influenced by others and who would never live with people I did not know. This independence set me apart in her eyes, and she shared how much she valued those traits.

Throughout my childhood, I frequently found myself in conflict with the boys in the family. Their wrestling matches and roughhousing unsettled me, and I would scream whenever they fought, convinced that someone would get hurt. Bea explained that this was typical behavior for boys and that they often teased me because my dislike of noise made me an easy target. She remembered how I would sit quietly behind doors, peeking out to observe, seeking peace and comfort away from the commotion.

Bea recognized my natural curiosity and desire to understand everything around me. Because of this, the boys did not tease me as much; they knew I was observant and had knowledge beyond my years. My quiet nature and preference for solitude made my place behind the door a refuge, and Bea understood this was where I felt most comfortable. She never saw a need to pull me out of my peaceful spot, knowing that I did not enjoy noise or constant company.

She also admitted that she didn't want Kathy and me to spend much time together because I lacked patience with her. Bea noted that spending time around Grandma Mae and living between two homes had made me wiser than expected for my age. She emphasized that I had developed a strong sense of judgment, always asking questions and showing an ability to sense when a person was good or not. In Bea's eyes, that trust and awareness set me apart from Kathy, who didn't share those same instincts and often found herself in risky situations.

Bea's Reflections on My Gifts and Identity

During one of our intimate conversations, Bea shared insights that left a lasting impression on me. She explained that the women in town were not afraid of me, but rather that they saw something mysterious within me—something unknown that unsettled them. Bea said that people often referenced my eyes, suggesting there was something unique about them that sparked curiosity and speculation.

Bea expressed disappointment that I had refused the gifts God had given me. She emphasized the importance of never rejecting what God offers, explaining that one day I would reach out to Him and ask for those gifts. She cautioned me never to tell God that I did not want a gift from Him, reinforcing the significance of accepting and embracing what is divinely bestowed.

In a moment of vulnerability, Bea revealed that she knew I smoked cigarettes to change the color of my eyes, hoping to conceal what she believed were God's gifts. Tears rolled down my face as I realized she was aware of my actions, and she gently confirmed it. Bea reassured me that it is impossible to hide what God wants to reveal and encouraged me to pray and give thanks, reminding me that I was chosen for a reason. She firmly believed that one day I would seek out the very gifts I had tried to suppress.

That night, I went to sleep with my arm around Bea, cherishing what I sensed might be our final moments together.

The next morning, my dad arrived early, and I witnessed one of the most cherished moments of my life—seeing two loved ones embrace forgiveness, peace, love, and respect.

Bea asked Shirley Jean to take Kathy with her to Milwaukee and place her in a center where she could seek help. I thought to myself, *I'm the one you sent to see a counselor. I'm the one who needs help.* But Bea wanted me to understand that her approach was rooted in her belief that I would be able to cope well after she was gone. She expressed confidence in my ability to navigate life's challenges and reassured me that she was not worried about the possibility of me making mistakes. Instead, she trusted in my capacity to learn, adapt, and recognize my own strengths over time. That trust was her way of encouraging my independence and personal growth.

I got into the bed with her as she began to show me all the nodules that had consumed her body. She told me the cancer had spread everywhere. I tried to say they were not cancer, but she would not hear me—she wanted me to understand the truth of what was happening to her.

A nurse entered the room to adjust her IV and brought a bag of plasma. Something went wrong, and the bag slipped, spilling over Bea and me. The nurse apologized and brought towels for us to clean up. Bea had so many things to tell me that day. Looking back, I understand she wasn't just talking—she wanted me to *feel* the reality of her illness and her body failing, even as I tried to deny it.

Bea's house and other relatives' homes were full, so Dad and I moved from place to place but continued visiting Bea's house to get updates from the older siblings, who managed the visiting schedule. Dad would go whenever he wanted, perhaps because there were differences in how things were handled between us younger siblings and the older ones. Meeting with the family gave us a sense of connection and kept us informed about Bea's condition, but waiting for a chance to visit her at the hospital was difficult because of the long lines of family members and friends who had known her for years.

David Lee's Family Meeting and the Prayer for Bea

My brother David Lee Curtis called a meeting with the family to address the reality of our mother's suffering. As we gathered, he began by acknowledging Bea's condition and the difficulty we all faced. David admitted that this was one of the hardest decisions he had ever made and expressed his hope that each of us could come together in understanding and acceptance.

The room was silent—so quiet it seemed no one dared to breathe. In that stillness, David spoke from the heart. He asked each of us to change our prayers: if Bea was not going to recover, we were to ask Father God to take her home and release her to His care. The weight of his words settled over all of us. I realized that this was one of the hardest prayers I had ever prayed. Letting go in faith and love challenged us deeply and marked a profound moment in our family's journey.

Bea's Final Moments with her besties, David Lee Curtis, Katie Lousie Curtis, Shirley Jean Curtis

Early the next morning, Shirley Jean called to say the doctor had advised her to notify the family that Bea would likely pass away by noon. My sister and her husband explained that they needed to inform their workplaces so we could visit Bea before she was gone.

Shirley Jean called what felt like every thirty minutes to let me know she was waiting for me. She told me, "Bea is holding on. She wants to see you." I felt like the world had moved from under my feet with no surface left to stand on. I told her I was waiting for my sister and her husband to return from work so I could go with them.

Later, Shirley Jean called again and said Bea had held on, waiting for her baby—but she was gone. Bea passed at exactly twelve o'clock noon.

When I finally understood that Bea had died at exactly noon, I was overcome with grief and a feeling of helplessness. I left the house and ran down the freeway, my eyes searching the sky as if hoping to see her one last time. Each breath felt surreal, as if I were floating in midair, disconnected from the ground beneath me. The loss left me exposed and vulnerable, longing for comfort in a moment that felt impossible to bear.

As I ran, I heard a car horn sounding behind me and then a familiar voice—my sister—asking where I was going. She eventually found me and confirmed Bea's passing. We both expressed deep regret that we had not arrived in time to say goodbye.

Afterward, I went to Blytheville, Arkansas, with my sister, her husband, and their children. Later, I returned to Chicago for about a month. By then, my brother Larry was living with Shirley Jean. He called to inform me that our sister needed help with her daughter and that she needed a caregiver to help her through the lengthy surgeries ahead. She would be in the hospital for quite some time. My job was in the process of transferring to Canada, but I decided instead to move to Milwaukee to take care of my sister—the same Shirley Jean who had helped Bea raise me.

I stayed close to two years. When I left, Shirley Jean was driving again and taking care of her household. I told her I needed to leave. I had a dream in which I saw someone with no leg and assumed it was me.

I later moved in with my sister, her husband, and their children again. Due to military orders, they relocated to San Bernardino, California. I was asked if I wanted to move with them. Our mother had insisted on it before she passed, and my sister, her husband, and one of my brothers all thought it would be good for me. I decided to go.

Bea's Quotes – In Her Words

1. Keep God first.

2. When God shows you someone, believe it.

3. Sudden visits make long friendships.

4. Choose your friends wisely.

5. You will always need a doctor, a lawyer, and an Indian chief.

6. Birds of a feather flock together.

7. "A man is breast and britches."

8. Don't forget where you come from; you might return there one day.

Chapter 13:
Warning Before the Storm

Upon my arrival in California, I focused on evaluating my mindset to determine the direction I wished to pursue. This period of self-reflection gave me the chance to carefully consider my options and identify the most promising path for my future. I visited several locations in the city and surrounding areas. While traveling in a nearby city, I noticed a sign that reminded me of my former job in Chicago.

I asked my sister if it was possible for me to check out the opportunities the company had to offer. I found that my experience and qualifications led to an immediate job offer that same day.

I found great satisfaction in handling key tasks at work, such as sorting components and completing iron wiring. These responsibilities were not only essential to the manufacturing process but also allowed me to demonstrate my attention to detail and commitment to quality. My proficiency in these areas did not go unnoticed; colleagues and supervisors began to suggest that I consider pursuing a career as a mechanic, recognizing the potential in my technical abilities.

I often heard about individuals who achieved success without attending college. During my formative years, technical schools were available, offering opportunities to acquire practical skills without spending several years in a traditional classroom setting. I have always found that my attention span is relatively short, which made alternative education paths particularly appealing to me.

I met a colleague at work who shared similar interests. We were the same age and both exploring potential career paths. She was a single parent of two children, and I was genuinely impressed by her ability to manage her household and maintain a nice vehicle. I was uncertain whether I would be willing or able to take on that much responsibility at this age. During my visits with her and the children, I observed that she managed the situation efficiently.

We often communicated by phone, despite her busy schedule. In a recent conversation, she invited me to join her at the club that evening. She lived outside the city.

My sister and her husband invited me to go with them to a club on the military post. I asked my sister if she would mind if my friend joined us at the club. She said yes, but preferred that my friend come over and ride with us. I called my friend, and she accepted.

The space was bustling, and there was a noticeable presence of many guys in attendance. Throughout the evening, we interacted with several individuals, exchanging contact information with those we connected with. This initial meeting led us to participate in their weekly events, allowing us to broaden our social circle and become more involved in the community.

I am generally more outgoing with strangers when I am alone. I tend to be reserved when meeting new people in the presence of friends. While identifying as a shy person, I have developed strategies to manage this tendency. The evening was enjoyable, so we agreed to visit frequently after seeing our acquaintance.

At present, I am not in a relationship, nor am I pursuing one. My primary focus is on self-discovery and developing a clearer understanding of my identity. Additionally, I am in the process of coping with Bea's passing and reflecting on how to move forward in her absence. I have not discussed her departure. Prior to her passing, our conversations led me to reflect on myself. She previously mentioned, "You'll have some bumps in the road, but you'll be fine," a comment that remains with me.

My friend called and asked if we could meet for lunch; she wanted to talk about technical schools outside the city. I accepted. We met at a pop-up restaurant and talked about our goals outside of work. I mentioned that I was looking for a technical school in the area but hadn't found one yet. I was concerned that college might not be suitable for me because I have difficulty maintaining attention for extended periods.

We both laughed as she observed that many individuals do not consider that aspect when thinking about college. She remarked that she had never previously viewed it from that perspective.

She then explained that most of the technical schools were in Rialto, California, which is a little over 30 minutes from San Bernardino, California.

During our conversation, my friend explained that there are numerous technical schools available, each designed to cater to different interests and career paths. This variety offers flexibility for individuals seeking alternatives to traditional college education. Personally, I was interested in pursuing Banking Operations, primarily because I wanted to strengthen my skills with numbers. When I mentioned this, my friend asked whether I was genuinely serious about the field. We shared a moment of laughter, as neither of us realized that the other was considering the same career direction.

My friend completed the required exam earlier that week and received her results—she successfully passed for the Banking Operations Technical School in Rialto, California. To mark this accomplishment, she invited me to join her in celebrating. She mentioned that she would be starting school in a few weeks and strongly recommended that I contact the school to schedule my own exam date so that I could begin the program as well.

She inquired about my proficiency with multiple-choice questions. I explained that I utilize the process of elimination effectively. She expressed confidence in my ability to pass the exam and mentioned that it typically requires approximately three hours to complete.

She provided the exam contact number and advised me to act promptly so I could begin with her. I called to schedule an appointment, received a date, and asked my sister to drive me to Rialto, California. I explained that the test would take about three hours. She stated she didn't mind; it would give her time to look around and check out some stores in the area.

About three days later, I received my exam results indicating that I had passed, and I was provided with a registration date. I contacted my friend to confirm if we had the same start date, as both of us needed to leave our jobs before beginning school.

My friend and I started school, which turned out to be more demanding than anticipated. After two weeks, I determined that prioritizing my studies was necessary.

The setup closely resembled that of a major banking institution, and my friend and I were impressed by the environment. About three weeks into the class, I noticed one classmate who consistently stood out from the rest. His confidence and unique approach to learning caught my attention, prompting me to reach out and spend more time with him. My goal was to observe his methods and gain valuable insights that might help me achieve my own academic objectives.

We quickly developed a routine of studying together, often dedicating substantial time to reviewing material and discussing concepts. Although he primarily served as my tutor rather than a fellow student needing to study, his guidance proved invaluable.

His willingness to help and depth of understanding made our study sessions both productive and motivating, providing me with much-needed support as I worked toward my goals.

I was impressed by his ability to come in, open, and close the bank without one penny being out of the equation. What a commanding presence. His example finally helped me understand things clearly. I called him my tutor. One evening after class, he said, "You don't need me. You just need to trust yourself. Stop second-guessing your knowledge—give yourself credit." I called my friend to share his thoughts.

During this period, my friend mistakenly assumed that I was interested in pursuing a relationship with the male student who stood out in class. She did not realize that I was having difficulty keeping up with the class material at the same pace as the other students, particularly the men. My interactions with him were primarily motivated by my efforts to improve academically, rather than any romantic interest. However, my friend thought I sometimes tended to exaggerate situations, often questioning whether I was making more out of things than necessary. She reminded me, "You passed the exam—that's why you're here." I welcomed her criticism. We became best friends, and I learned to enjoy my weekends.

One day, I received an unexpected phone call from Barbara Robinson- Hunts, a friend from back home whom I had not spoken to since moving to California. She shared that she had recently visited my oldest sister Katie residence in Mississippi and, during her visit, had asked for my contact information. Barbara wanted to check in and see how I was doing, expressing her concern after having a dream in which she saw me experiencing significant weight loss. Although I reassured her that I do not have any issues with my weight and did not quite understand the meaning of her dream at the time, I admitted that stress sometimes affects my appetite, making me less likely to eat during challenging periods.

We continued our conversation, and I told Barbara how wonderful it was to hear from her after so long. I explained that I was currently attending school and that everything was going well for me. At this point in my journey, I felt much more comfortable and confident, finally feeling that I truly belonged in my class.

On a pleasant and sunny day spent with my sister, I observed a distinctive vehicle I had previously seen in another state. I suggested that we knew him from the base we left before arriving here. We were only acquainted with him through mutual friends. My sister observed that these types of cars are prevalent worldwide. I replied that we often saw this vehicle, and thinking it belonged to someone familiar, I suggested following it to confirm. My sister agreed.

We arrived simultaneously at our destination, exchanged cordial laughter, and received parking instructions. The individual greeted us enthusiastically, despite our status as acquaintances with shared mutual friends. He, along with his associates from the last post, held considerable popularity both on and off base. My sister extended a dinner invitation, which he accepted.

As we left, I told my sister he was just an acquaintance, not a friend. We had seen him at the base club and around the base. I recounted an occasion when our niece Shelia visited the military base where we previously resided. I reminded my sister about dropping us off at a club and later attending an after-party at his residence. To help her remember, I provided details about his social connections and regular interactions with different individuals in town. We frequently saw him at the grocery store on Sundays with different women. She joked about me pursuing him, but I noted his reputation with women. During our attendance at his house party, we exchanged polite smiles as I observed his active social interactions from a distance.

He arrived for dinner, and we discussed mutual acquaintances. As time passed, we spent increasing amounts of time together and formed a relationship. He was only there for school, which lasted about several months, and then he would return to his duty assignment.

Time seemed to pass quickly, and before we knew it, months in the program had come to an end. He completed the course with ease, not needing to devote extra time to studying, and successfully passed without difficulty. As graduation drew near, he expressed his wish for me to attend the ceremony in support of his achievement.

I fully intended to be present at his graduation; however, during this period, I began to experience serious health problems. These issues escalated, and I was subsequently admitted to the hospital, which prevented me from attending the event as planned.

He visited me at the hospital on the night of his graduation, filled with excitement. He is intelligent, possesses a wonderful sense of humor, and is always full of laughter. He often spoke about his grandmother and the profound impact she had on his life; the stories he shared reflected his deep admiration for her, and his face would light up whenever he mentioned her. The words she used reminded me of Bea, and we would laugh together at her expressions, which was a quality I greatly appreciated in him. He graduated with impressive ease, retaining information effortlessly—a skill I truly admired. Although I wished I could have celebrated with him, I was genuinely happy for his achievements. I encouraged him to celebrate with his classmates, knowing that he would soon be leaving after graduation. We made plans for me to visit him once I completed my own course and even discussed the possibility of marriage and me relocating to be with him. After a couple of days, he left; however, we maintained daily communication to discuss our future.

I returned to school after my time in the hospital. It was getting close to the end. My friend and I were approaching the completion of our course and were looking forward to new opportunities ahead. The male friend who had tutored me recently started joining us for lunch and various events around town. This was a change from my usual routine, as I typically spent lunchtime in class studying. I told my friend I might be leaving once I graduated, and my best friend thought it would be good if I secured a job there first, especially since the school offered positions after graduation; she felt that I might want to take that into consideration. It seemed like things were moving in the right direction. We had at least five to six weeks before graduation.

We got a call from family members in Los Angeles, California requesting that we join them for the holiday weekend for a pool party and barbecue. My family decided to attend the gathering. At the time, I didn't feel physically ill, but I had an unusual sense that something wasn't quite right. During the visit, my aunt Odessa approached me and asked if I was feeling okay. I assured her that I was fine, but for the first time, she expressed concern about my appearance—specifically, my eyes. She remarked that my eyes seemed to have a strange look and wanted to know if I truly felt well. Once again, I responded that I felt fine, even though I was beginning to wonder about her observations.

After enjoying a wonderful weekend and spending time with my family, even though I felt sluggish and not quite like myself, I knew something was wrong. What it was, I did not know. Maybe it was the medication—I just knew I wasn't my usual self. We left for the two-hour drive back to San Bernardino on Sunday.

When we arrived home, the kids were filled with excitement, eagerly sharing how much fun they had at the beach and describing their walk to the forum. Everyone enjoyed the stroll together, and it was clear that the outing had been a memorable experience for all of us. As the evening settled in, I was mindful that school would resume on Monday, so I took the time to unwind. After getting home, I took a bath, relaxed, and eventually went to bed, falling asleep with thoughts of the wonderful weekend and the joy of seeing my cousins. Listening to the kids enthusiastically recount the highlights of our trip reminded me of how special these family moments are.

Chapter 14: Chosen Cancer

I woke up for school that morning feeling mostly okay—just a little tired, maybe from the trip. My friend picked me up, as she often did, since I lived closer to the school than she did. It was a busy morning in class, and by lunchtime my girlfriend and I decided to go out to eat. My friend—the one who tutored me— asked if he could join us. We went to a restaurant not far from school.

After returning, we went back to our booth on campus. As soon as I sat down, I jumped up quickly. I felt a sharp, pointed pinch in my rectum, like sudden pressure or something lodged there. I shifted around in the chair, trying to figure out what it was, but the sensation didn't go away.

When I got home, I told my sister what I was feeling. She suggested I probably needed a laxative. I had never used one before and didn't really know much about them, but I decided to follow her recommendation. We went to the pharmacy and bought a laxative.

The next day, I returned to school. The sharp sensation came back again, as if something were stuck in my rectum. The discomfort was so intense that I had to stand up, but even standing didn't relieve the pressure. It affected both sitting and standing. I moved from side to side for the rest of class, just trying to get through it.

After school, I told my sister that I needed to see a doctor. It was clear something was wrong and wasn't going away on its own, so we went to the emergency room. Being new to the area, I felt it was important to get checked.

The hospital we went to—San Bernardino Hospital—was a Catholic hospital not far from our home. On **August 23, 1982**, I presented there with severe lower back pain, abdominal pain, and a fever of 102°F. After examining me, the physician told me I had an infection in one of my fallopian tubes. He prescribed antibiotics and scheduled a follow-up appointment in approximately two weeks.

After taking the medication for about three doses, I began to decline instead of improve. I was vomiting, extremely weak, and could barely stand.

My sister contacted the physician, who advised her to take me back to the emergency room. After more tests, the surgeon said I would need a minor surgical procedure—a "bikini incision"—to find out what was really going on.

Following the surgery, the doctor diagnosed an infection in my tubes. I remained in the hospital for several days, and when I was discharged, I was told to go to the pharmacy for more antibiotics. I went home with my medication, hoping recovery was just a matter of time.

But within a few days at home, I noticed swelling and knew I wasn't improving. I was still weak, feverish, and vomiting. I ended up sitting on the bathroom floor, too weak to stand. My sister found me there, helped me back to bed, and called the surgeon again. He told her to bring me back to the hospital immediately.

When we arrived in the emergency room, the surgeon was already waiting for me. After additional tests, he concluded that I needed a hysterectomy.

I resisted the idea. I wanted to postpone the surgery until after I had children. The doctor told me there was no time for that—that waiting was not an option. It was an incredibly painful moment. The possibility that I might never have children was devastating. My mother had twelve children, and all my siblings were parents. I couldn't understand why I was in this position.

MY sister Missie, sister-in-law Eva and the doctor continued discussing the situation while I struggled to process it. The swelling and constant pain made everything feel heavier. Being in a Catholic hospital, I knew a hysterectomy would only be performed if it was considered medically necessary. That alone told me how serious things were.

I wasn't getting better, and eventually I accepted that I had no real choice. I agreed to have the surgery, thinking this was the worst thing that could possibly happen to me.

After surgery, it's standard practice for the surgeon to visit and explain the results. But I didn't see **Dr. Luke Hsiao** after the procedure—not once. I requested to speak with him, but days passed and there was still no update.

While I was recovering, my sister came to visit, bringing her husband and my sister-in-law. I noticed that my brother-in-law's face looked swollen, and I asked him what happened. I also wondered why he was there at all, since he was supposed to be away at military school for several months. He said he had fallen at school and that the fall caused the swelling, but he reassured me he was okay.

My sister-in-law was wearing sunglasses. We talked, and I told them I still hadn't seen Dr. Hsiao—not even once—since the surgery, even though it's routine for surgeons to check in on their patients afterwards.

They said maybe he had come by while I was asleep and didn't want to wake me. I pointed out that he had woken me up before on previous visits. They encouraged me to get some rest and assured me the doctor would come soon. After a few hours, they left to check on the kids and get food.

Once they were gone, I fell asleep. At some point, a woman entered my room. She started talking about things that didn't make sense to me, and she quickly realized I was confused. She asked if I had spoken with my doctor. I told her no. She then asked if my family had spoken to me about the surgery. Again, I said no.

I told her that I wanted to speak with my doctor. She placed a card on the table beside my bed and said she would come back after my family and surgeon had talked with me.

When she left, I felt a strong sense that something wasn't right. My mother had always told me to pay attention to those quiet inner nudges—that the spirit speaks softly, not loudly, and that I needed to listen. I felt prompted to pick up the card.

I looked at it, but I didn't understand what it meant. The words on it confused me. That same inner prompting led me to dial the number written on the card.

When I called, a woman answered, and the name she used to identify the office didn't connect with anything I understood at the time. I asked her politely, "Ma'am, could you please repeat the word you just used when you answered the phone?" She went quiet. I explained that someone from her office had visited me, but I didn't understand what they were talking about. I asked her to explain what their business was, and what the words on the card meant—for someone who didn't know.

I remember her explanation in my own words:

"Terminally ill cancer patients have cancers that cannot be cured. Treatment is focused on improving comfort and, when possible, increasing life expectancy."

I screamed and dropped the phone. Hospital staff rushed into the room, trying to calm me down. I cried out, asking them to please have **Dr. Hsiao** come see me. They told me they had already paged him and that he was on his way. They also said my family had been contacted and were on their way to the hospital. Dr. Hsiao had prescribed something to help me relax, but I refused it. I wanted to keep my mind clear.

I don't know how long it took before **Dr. Luke Hsiao** came into the room, but when he did, I was crying uncontrollably. He tried to comfort me. I asked him, "Why didn't you come see me after surgery?"

He told me he was sorry. I asked him, "What happened to me?"

He started to explain and said, "I'm sorry," again. My family had arrived by then. He leaned across the foot of my bed and began to cry, repeating, "I've tried so hard, but the cancer is severe and there's nothing I can do." He said it more than once.

I felt shattered. I had already endured two procedures. Then I was told I needed a hysterectomy. Now I was being told I had *terminal cancer* and no treatment options. At my age, it felt impossible to bear. I wondered: Was anyone ever going to tell me I was dying?

My sister later told me that Dr. Hsiao had told the family he couldn't bring himself to tell me, and had asked them to share the news—but they hadn't been able to, either.

I could see that Dr. Hsiao was as disturbed by the situation as I was. He had done all he could, and there was nothing more he could offer medically. I found myself feeling compassion for him too, even in my own shock.

He suggested prescribing medication to help with my stress. I told him I didn't want it and that I preferred to be alone. I told the staff that if I decided I needed something, I would let the nurse know. I asked them to close the blinds, turn off the television, and let me have silence.

Once the room was dark and quiet, I curled into the fetal position and let the weight of everything wash over me.

I remembered when my sister's baby died in that house fire, from smoke inhalation. I had asked Bea why my sister's baby had died, and Bea told me the baby went to be with God. She reminded me back then that everyone is born to die—that death is inescapable. That truth had stayed with me, even affecting my sleep as a child.

Now I found myself asking Bea, in my spirit, why I had been placed in a situation that would end in my own death. I told her that if I'd been given a choice, I wouldn't have come, knowing this would be the outcome.

Bea always used to say, "You come into this world alone, and you will leave alone." In my spirit, I was now having a conversation with her and with God.

I remembered asking Bea, before she passed, to talk to God on my behalf. I remembered her saying that Madea had arrived for her, and how I could hear her talking with her.

Now, in that hospital bed, I asked Bea to please ask God if He would bring me through, the way He brought her through in her own time.

I prayed:

God, please help me through this. Help me face my fears and this uncertainty.

I must have fallen asleep resting in what I call Bea's "womb"— that deep comfort I felt when I thought of her. At that moment, I didn't feel like I had any tasks left to complete. What weighed on me most was my dad. I wanted to talk to him. I felt that everyone else would somehow manage if I were gone, but my absence would hurt him deeply. I remembered him telling me that he would stand in Bea's place for me, knowing how much I needed her and how these challenges would have pulled her to my side no matter what.

Every time I slept, I began to dream of places I didn't recognize. I wondered if they represented something about life or death, though I had no idea what death truly felt like. The strangest part was that I didn't *feel* like I was dying. Physically, aside from the weakness and weight loss, I still felt like myself. I kept thinking: *If I have terminal cancer, why does everything still feel the same?*

I remembered how Bea, when her lung cancer had spread to her bones, would show me the nodules all over her body. She would guide my hand so I could feel the small lumps. I told her they weren't cancer. She insisted they were. She wasn't sad; she accepted the reality even as she wasn't ready to go. She had no choice but to accept her fate.

It pained my soul to think of how strong Bea had been, yet how exhausted she looked near the end. I saw a woman who never truly got to know the love of a man in a lasting, faithful way. That saddened me deeply. So many of the men in her life—including my dad—struggled with alcohol. Dad didn't fully realize how much he loved Bea until he saw her lying in a hospital bed, the same woman who had held the household together after he left. She held everything in place.

Sitting in my own hospital bed on **September 23, 1982**, at around 4:30 p.m., I felt helpless.

I didn't see much of Dr. Hsiao around that time. I assumed there was nothing more he could do for me and that he was probably focusing on patients he could help. What I didn't know was that he was searching around the world looking for a patient who has survive my type of cancer—people who had survived at least a year and were in remission.

Having grown up on and around military bases since I was fifteen, I had seen my share of hardship. Now, with this cancer diagnosis, I still felt strangely as if there was nothing wrong with me—or maybe this was just what the beginning of the end felt like.

On a Friday evening, **Dr. Luke Hsiao** entered my room with my family. It was a moment I will never forget. Once everyone settled in, he began to share a story about another doctor whose patient had been diagnosed with the same type of cancer I had. Remarkably, that patient was doing well and was currently in remission.

I asked him for more details. He explained that this patient had gone through a full year of treatment and was now considered cancer-free in remission. For the first time since my diagnosis, I felt a flicker of real hope.

Dr. Hsiao told us he had spoken with the surgeon and his team who had treated that patient. Together, we began to discuss a plan for me to pursue the same opportunity.

I asked where this doctor was located, and Dr. Hsiao said, "UCLA—about two hours from San Bernardino." I asked, assuming it was just a college, "So I'm going to a school?" He explained that UCLA was not just a college—it was one of the most advanced hospitals in the world.

He said the doctor's name was **Dr. Neville Hacker**, a world-renowned specialist in this type of cancer. He told me that Dr. Hacker and his team were waiting for me.

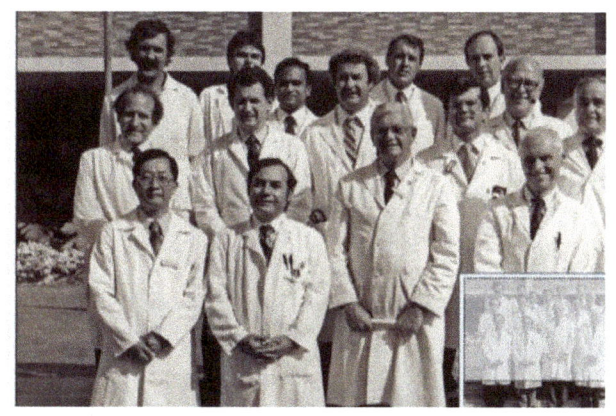

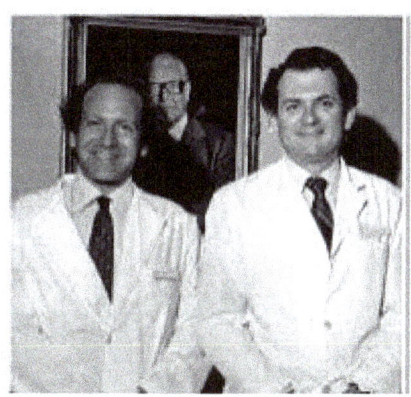

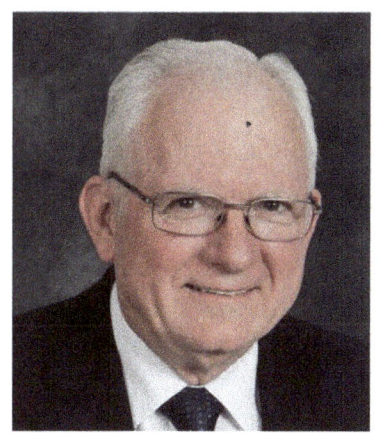

I asked about my stitches. "Are they going to open the same incision again?" I had just had surgery and was worried about going through it again so soon. He confirmed that yes, they would be reopening the same wound.

I told him I felt weak, that I had lost so much weight, and that I didn't know if my body could handle another surgery.

He looked at me and said, "There's a talented team of people waiting for you, and they are very good at what they do."

After discussing everything with Dr. Hsiao and my family, they all agreed it was worth trying. Their support helped me say yes. I told him I didn't want to travel there by ambulance. My sister offered to drive if he approved, and he did. I asked him if he really thought I could handle the ride, and he told me he wouldn't allow it if he didn't believe I could.

I asked when I had to be there. He said my check-in was scheduled for **Sunday**. With that, the preparations began.

Saturday was busy. Hospital staff came in and out, making sure everything was in order for the transfer. I spent that time reflecting on so much—on Bea, on that little girl behind the door who never felt fully protected, on the older women who seemed afraid of my eyes, on the gift Bea said I had.

Bea once told me I could see things before they happened. At the time, I didn't want that gift. She warned me that one day I would regret rejecting it and would ask God to give it back. She believed I was chosen for something I didn't fully understand.

Reflections on the Gift

At one point, my niece Charleetra Johnson Horne (Lisa) was curious about the abilities she had heard discussed within our family. She approached her aunt, my sister Shirley Jean, and asked how I was able to perceive things before they happened—if I truly possessed such a gift. In response, Shirley Jean explained that she was born with this gift but had always chosen not to embrace it. She, much like Bea, believed that accepting and understanding these abilities would happen naturally, in their own time. This perspective brought a measure of comfort and patience to our family's experience with the unknown, assuring us that acceptance was a journey rather than a forced decision.

Bea told me she treated me differently because she recognized my abilities early. She was disappointed that I feared the gift, and she suspected some of that fear came from how older women in town reacted to me. I know there is something unique about me, something many people don't see. My mind often runs at night, replaying faces and moments from my time at San Bernardino Hospital. I'm learning patience with myself and with the process of understanding these things.

Since I arrived at this hospital, I've been treated with respect. Their care supported me through some of the most difficult days of my life. Now, tomorrow, my journey would continue—to UCLA.

On **Sunday afternoon, October 2, 1982**, we finished packing. Dr. Luke Hsiao personally oversaw my departure from San Bernardino Hospital, making sure I had everything I needed for the trip and that I would be comfortable. As I rolled out of that hospital, I stayed strong outside, determined to face whatever came.

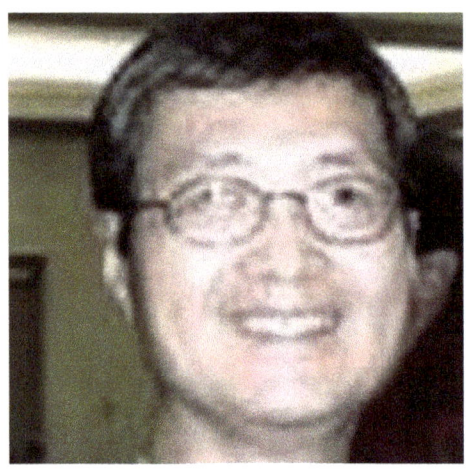

Throughout my stay at San Bernardino Hospital, Dr. Hsiao referred to me as "Little Girl." Though it was a simple nickname, it carried significant meaning for me. In moments when I felt most vulnerable and uncertain about my future, this small gesture conveyed a genuine tenderness and compassion. It was not just a casual phrase; it was an acknowledgment of my fears and struggles, offered with warmth and understanding.

Dr. Hsiao's concern and kindness helped ease my sense of isolation, making it easier for me to endure such a challenging time. His unwavering belief in seeking another solution for my condition gave me hope when I most needed it. Even when the path forward seemed out of touch, his persistence in finding hope was remarkable. Through his actions and words, Dr. Hsiao played a pivotal role in changing the course of my story, reminding me that I was not alone and that there was still a reason to hope.

As I left San Bernardino that day, I stepped into the unknown. Despite my fears, I did not leave without hope—thanks in large part to the compassion and determination Dr. Hsiao showed me throughout my journey.

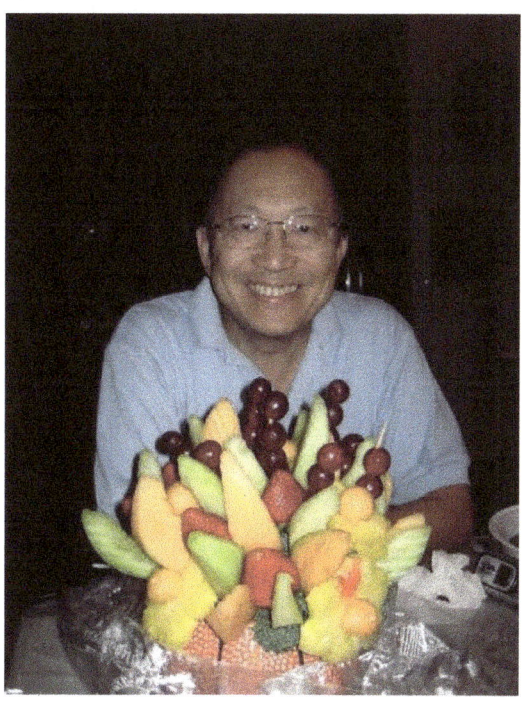

Chapter 15:
Part 1 — Welcome to UCLA

The journey from San Bernardino to UCLA was filled with anticipation and uncertainty. As we traveled through unfamiliar streets, I became increasingly aware of the emotional significance of leaving behind those who had supported me during such a difficult time. The staff at San Bernardino Hospital had become a source of stability and comfort, and the idea of beginning a new chapter was both daunting and hopeful.

Arriving at UCLA marked the beginning of a new phase in my treatment and recovery. The transition brought challenges, but it also held the possibility of healing. Everything was unfamiliar, and the future was unknown, yet I was determined to face whatever came next with courage. The encouraging words from Dr. Luke Hsiao strengthened my resolve, reminding me that I was not alone. With hope and resilience, I prepared myself for this next step, trusting the care that awaited me and believing in the possibility of survival.

We reached California in the early evening, but finding the hospital proved more difficult than expected. After driving around, retracing our path, and trying to follow directions, we finally located the hospital and felt immediate relief. Everyone agreed to stop for burgers and fries, ordering food to go so we could eat once I was settled in.

We arrived at UCLA on Sunday evening—an experience I will never forget. Although we had been assured that preparations were made for my arrival, it quickly became clear that everything was *not* ready. This unexpected situation made me question whether I truly belonged there.

While waiting for the admission process to finish, my sister and sister-in-law encouraged me to eat, but I chose to wait until I reached my room. My hesitation came from my experience at San Bernardino Hospital, where eating caused severe nausea and vomiting, leaving me extremely weak.

The check-in process was long, partly due to the complexity of my medical history. Once I was admitted and changed into the hospital gown the nurse provided, she told me that Dr. Hacker was aware I had arrived and would see me after meeting with his team. After getting settled, I finally decided to eat something—just as I expected, the nausea came within fifteen minutes. Soon after, I vomited.

My sister and sister-in-law immediately came to my aid, gently cleaning me up and helping me back into bed after the episode of nausea and vomiting. Despite their care, I remained extremely weak, and the nausea only continued to worsen. Concerned about my well-being, they reached out to the nurse's station for help. Unfortunately, the nurses informed them that no medication could be administered until the doctor arrived, leaving me with little option but to wait in discomfort.

They stayed by my side for as long as possible, offering comfort and support during this difficult transition. However, their responsibilities eventually called them away—they needed to prepare their children for school, and the drive home was at least an hour and a half. Before leaving, they embraced me and offered words of reassurance, promising that I would be okay. They also made sure to ask the nursing staff to have the doctor contact them with updates about my condition, ensuring I would not be left entirely alone as I faced the night ahead.

During this painful time, my boyfriend became an emotional anchor for me. He called day and night to check on me, sent flowers, cards, and letters—giving me strength to hold on when everything around me felt uncertain. Even from a distance, his support helped me keep fighting.

I have often kept certain struggles between myself and God. I didn't want to show my vulnerability. After my family left, I felt that whatever I was facing was between me and God alone. I needed to understand—not "Why me?" but *What do You know about me that I don't know?*

It was Sunday evening when I heard a knock on the door. A man with the most unique voice I had ever heard stepped inside. Only God could have chosen such a voice for this moment. He asked if they could come in, and I said yes. Several men in white coats entered the room behind him. He spoke first:

"Hello, I am Dr. Neville Hacker. Welcome to UCLA."

Each doctor then introduced himself. Tears formed in my eyes—sadness, fear, and loneliness all rising at once. They could see I was overwhelmed. Dr. Hacker spoke gently.

"We understand you experienced vomiting and nausea after eating. How are you feeling now?"

"It goes away once everything comes up," I answered.

He asked who brought me to the hospital. I explained that my sister and sister-in-law had driven me, but had to leave to get their children ready for school.

He asked about my mother.

"She's deceased—lung cancer that spread to the bone. Two years ago."

He asked about my father.

"He's in Mississippi. Because of his hearing impairment, involving him might cause frustration for both of us."

He asked whether my family had been informed about my condition.

"Yes," I answered.

"And who is the decision-maker concerning your treatment here?"

"Me."

He confirmed whether I understood that survival might not be possible.

"Yes," I said. "Dr. Hsiao told me."

The doctors appeared concerned. I became emotional again, feeling alone. Dr. Hacker could sense my fear and helplessness.

He asked, "May I examine you?"

"Yes," I agreed, though fear gripped me—being examined by a room full of white men in white coats was overwhelming for a young Black girl from Mississippi. Yet I remained still.

The examination was remarkable. Dr. Hacker used his fingers to identify the size of the tumors in my vagina and rectum. The other doctors observed and took notes. Hearing him describe the sizes with such precision, I felt confirmation from God: *This is where you are supposed to be.*

Afterward, he asked, "Are you a person of faith?"

"Yes, I believe in God."

"That's important," he said. "Because we're going to need Him."

His words will stay with me forever.

He asked whom I wanted him to update on my progress.

"MYSELF," I said loudly.

The doctors smiled, and Dr. Hacker replied, "We will honor your preferences."

I explained why: the first time I was diagnosed, no one told me. They asked who eventually delivered the news. I told them about the woman who had stopped by my room. She left a card, and it was only when I called the number that I learned the truth—I was terminal.

Dr. Hacker asked how everything began. I explained:

It had started as a wonderful day. I was close to graduating, excited about my future in Banking Operations. I had lunch with classmates. When I returned and sat down, I suddenly felt something sharp in my rectum. Standing relieved it a little, but the pressure didn't stop. My sister thought it was constipation, though I had never experienced that. The laxative didn't work. I had no pain—just the feeling that something was stuck. Eventually, I needed hospitalization and two surgeries, which led me here.

The team explained that the questions were needed due to the seriousness of my illness.

Cancer affects not only the body but also the mind and spirit. The diagnosis had shaken me emotionally—fear, sadness, confusion, uncertainty about the future. The support of family and the medical team was essential.

One of the white-coat doctors stayed by my bed, speaking to me gently while Dr. Hacker and the others reviewed notes. They returned to my bedside together.

"You now have the support of a family here," they said.

Dr. Hacker ordered nausea medication and encouraged me to rest. They said they would return the next day with more information about my surgery date and time.

Chapter 15:
Part 2 — Welcome to UCLA:
Return to My Mother's Womb

The night before surgery, an overwhelming need for comfort came over me, pulling me into a fetal position—as if I were back in my mother's womb. I whispered that the doctors had told me there was a chance I might not survive. I feared that meant I was going to die. In that moment, I remembered how you, Bea, had always prepared me for moments like this—teaching me about Jesus, God, and crossing over. I remembered hearing you speak to Madea when you were nearing the end of your own life.

I admitted my fear of dying and asked you to speak to God on my behalf, to help bring me through this. As I cried, something in my mind and body aligned perfectly. A deep warmth, like a blanket of peace, wrapped around me. It was a kind of safety I hadn't felt in years—like I had been allowed to return to the sanctuary of my mother's womb.

As sleep settled over me, something extraordinary happened. I felt myself drifting out of my body, weightless and calm. A gentle voice echoed in my spirit, repeating the same reassuring words:

"You are healed. Wake up. They're going in to clean you."

The words dissolved my fear. I felt as though I was moving on autopilot. Guided by something greater than myself, I stood up, walked to the bathroom, and gently covered my prior surgical incision with my hand. I couldn't feel my feet on the ground. It felt as though I were being carried.

I cleaned myself with a quiet sense of calm. There was no logical explanation—only a feeling that God was guiding each movement.

Almost instinctively, I reached for my makeup bag and began to apply makeup, preparing myself as if for an important event.

Suddenly, a loud scream shattered the silence. When I opened the bathroom door, my sister, Missie, and my sister-in-law, Eva, were both staring at me with shock on their faces—pale, frozen, as if they had seen a ghost. Their reaction made me pause and question how I had gotten into the bathroom, and why I had chosen to put on makeup before major surgery.

They kept pleading, "Please don't leave the hospital—please don't leave."

Confused, I finally answered, "I'm getting ready for surgery."

Both of them frantically asked, "Why do you have on makeup? You can't wear makeup to surgery."

I looked at myself. A voice within me answered:

"This is how I see myself."

Just as they tried to convince me to remove it, there was a knock at the door.

"Good morning—we're here to take you to surgery."

The very first thing they said was that the makeup had to come off. I begged them not to remove it. One of them called Dr. Hacker.

He stepped into my room, took one look at me, and said gently:

"She looks beautiful. Aww...okay. Let her keep it on."

Dr. Hacker understood what others missed—that keeping my makeup on wasn't vanity. It was identity. It was courage. It was the last expression of myself before facing life or death. It gave me grounding, strength, and dignity. His kindness gave me the reassurance I needed to walk into the unknown.

Dr. Hacker's Compassion and the Surgical Plan

From the beginning, Dr. Hacker explained everything with clarity and compassion. He went through my diagnosis, my lab results, and every treatment option. He made complex medical information easy to understand, leaving no room for confusion or fear. His goal was to pursue every trace of cancer—to go after all of it—and he made sure I understood each step we took.

The surgery would be long—possibly lasting from morning until late at night. After every incision, a biopsy would be performed. They could not move forward until each biopsy was read. It was exhausting just to think about.

Having already gone through two surgeries, I feared my body wouldn't survive another one.

When I asked if I would make it through, Dr. Hacker looked at me with confidence and said:

"You can handle it. It won't be a problem."

His certainty became my strength.

Recovery: ICU and the Return to Life

I lost track of how long I stayed in the ICU; the days and nights seemed to blur together in an endless haze. The constant hum of machines and the dim lighting made it impossible to distinguish one hour from the next.

My sense of time faded, replaced by an intense focus on healing and survival. The hours and days blurred together, leaving me uncertain of how long I had been in the ICU. Amidst this haze, Dr. Hacker entered quietly and gently woke me with a warm smile. His reassuring presence immediately put me at ease, bringing calm to the chaos.

With genuine happiness, Dr. Hacker shared the news I had longed to hear: "We got it—all the cancer." As his words sank in, relief and gratitude washed over me. I realized that the exhausting ordeal had led to a hopeful outcome, and I began to process the meaning of this moment—knowing that, against immense odds, there was now a path forward.

When I finally moved to my room, I was overwhelmed by the flowers and cards my boyfriend had sent. Later that evening, Dr. Hacker came to check on me. Seeing the flowers made him smile—he knew I needed all the support I could get.

The number of tubes attached to me frightened me. One tube, they explained, connected directly to my heart. I had two private-duty nurses. My night nurse was deeply spiritual—she prayed over me every time I moved. She read the Bible for hours, rubbing my hand gently as if comforting a child.

As my body slowly healed, the team suggested counseling because of everything I had endured at such a young age. Every day a tube or device was removed. I began asking questions about each machine, each sound, each tube. One device—a suction machine on my left—caught my attention.

Introduction to the Fecal Management System (FMS)

The FMS is used to manage stool for patients who may not need a permanent colostomy. One morning, two women entered with supplies, asking me to roll to my right. Confused, I asked what they were doing.

They were following the doctor's orders, but I panicked. Overcome with emotion, I begged them to call Dr. Hacker before doing anything. Through tears, I pleaded that I believed in God's healing and didn't need the bags.

A Compassionate Conversation with Dr. Hacker

Dr. Hacker entered the room, exuding a sense of calm and patience. His understanding demeanor immediately helped to ease my anxiety. After assessing the situation, he gently asked the nurses to remove the supplies and step out, giving us a moment of privacy.

Once we were alone, Dr. Hacker took the time to explain the purpose of the device. He described why it was likely necessary for my recovery, ensuring I understood its role in my healing process. Sensing my apprehension, he reassured me that we could revisit this conversation later, allowing me the space to process and ask questions when I felt ready.

My Secret Battle with the Machine

After Dr. Hacker left, my focus shifted back to the suction machine by my side. Driven by curiosity and a quiet determination, I carefully pulled the device closer to me. With a mixture of apprehension and resolve, I reached over and turned it off. Almost immediately, a wave of nausea swept over me, accompanied by the unpleasant taste of stool in my mouth. Alarmed, I quickly switched the machine back on.

Still, I was not ready to give up. I began to test my limits, experimenting in secret. First, I left the machine off for just one minute—then, after seeing how my body reacted, I waited five minutes, then thirty, and eventually an hour. This became my private ritual, something I kept entirely to myself, not sharing it with anyone—not my nurses, not even Dr. Hacker.

Ever since the morning of my surgery, when I was abruptly awakened by that mysterious voice, I had felt an invisible force guiding me through my recovery. I could not explain what it was, but it gave me strength and a sense of purpose as I navigated each new challenge.

The Breakthrough

One day, Dr. Hacker returned and told me he would be turning off the device so my body could function naturally. He needed to confirm whether my intestines were working.

When he turned it off, the silence was overwhelming.

He asked if I felt nauseated.

"No," I answered.

"That's a good sign," he said.

He reminded me that I needed to have a bowel movement. If successful, he could remove the tube from my side.

Later, after lunch, I allowed myself to relax on the commode. Something inside told me not to strain, just breathe. A peaceful calm settled over me—and then, finally, my body responded naturally.

Tears filled my eyes.

I pulled the nurse's cord. When she entered, she found me crying. She asked if I needed help standing. I told her no. When she saw the commode, she immediately notified Dr. Hacker and the staff.

They entered the room rejoicing.

Dr. Hacker smiled—everyone did.

It was a victory. A miracle. A turning point.

He told me to keep eating, and if I maintained progress for a few more days, he would remove the tube. That night, I couldn't wait to tell my night nurse. When she arrived, Bible in hand, I shared the news and we prayed together until I fell asleep.

A Breath of Fresh Air

The next morning, one of the nurses approached me with a gentle suggestion. She asked if I would like to go downstairs to a seating area—a spot where I could watch people coming and going. The simple idea of leaving my room, feeling fresh air on my skin and sunlight warming my face, felt like a promise of freedom and renewal.

With her help, I carefully got dressed, and together we made our way to the first floor. As I sat there, watching all the students moving in and out of the hospital—home, choosing to sit outside among us—I experienced a new perspective. This moment gave me a sense of wanting to remain present, to embrace the now. Life beyond what once seemed impossible began to feel like a future within reach.

Anticipating Discharge: Emotions and Gratitude

Dr. Hacker explained that if I continued to show progress, I would soon be discharged from the hospital. This news stirred a complex mix of emotions within me. On the one hand, there was happiness at the thought of moving forward in my recovery, but on the other, a sense of sadness at the prospect of leaving behind the people who had become so important to me.

The staff and caregivers who had supported me were more than just medical professionals—they had become like family during my time in the hospital. Everyone, including psychologists, therapists, nurses, and doctors, contributed significantly to my healing and sense of renewal. Their encouragement and care made a profound impact on my journey.

I truly believed that God had placed each member of this team in my life at exactly the right moment, using their dedication to strengthen both my mind and my spirit. Their presence was a constant source of hope and comfort as I prepared to take the next step toward recovery.

Chemotherapy: The Battle Within

Once I was discharged from the hospital, my journey was far from over. The next phase involved six months of chemotherapy—a challenge that quickly proved to be the hardest battle of my life.

The Physical and Emotional Toll

The memory of my first treatment remains vivid. I recall the initial pinch of the needle, followed by a strange, metallic taste in my mouth. This marked the beginning of a difficult ordeal. Almost immediately, dizziness swept over me, leaving me feeling unsettled and vulnerable. Among the various medications administered, one was known to affect less than one percent of patients worldwide. Yet, I was among that small group, which added another layer of uncertainty and fear to the process.

Loss and Vulnerability

The second chemotherapy treatment brought another harsh reality: the sudden loss of my hair. It happened unexpectedly while my sister-in-law Eva was shampooing my hair. She panicked as she saw my hair come away in a single cap, falling into my hands. The shock of seeing myself like this stripped away the sense of normalcy I had tried to hold onto. Underneath, I was left with fine hair, reminiscent of a newborn baby.

Strength Tested

Before starting chemotherapy, I felt strong—resilient and prepared to face whatever lay ahead. However, after each treatment, I felt increasingly destroyed and weakened. The stark difference between my sense of strength before and the exhaustion after each session was both painful and confusing, leaving me to grapple with the reality of my changing body and spirit.

Seeking Comfort

During my fourth treatment, overwhelmed by the physical and emotional toll, I turned to God in prayer. In the midst of my struggle, I sought comfort and understanding, hoping to find solace and strength to persevere.

"You healed me. Why am I taking something that makes me sick?"

Choosing Faith Over Chemotherapy

After deep prayer and reflection, I called UCLA and asked to speak with Dr. Hacker. I told him I would not be returning for more chemotherapy. I believed God had healed me.

Dr. Hacker already knew how strong that conviction was. Over the phone, in a gentle voice, he asked if I would consider one more treatment. After that, he said, the three of us—God, him, and me—could "shake hands" and agree to move forward.

Choosing Faith Over Chemotherapy

After spending time in deep prayer and reflection, I reached out to UCLA asking to speak directly with Dr. Hacker. With resolve in my voice, I explained to him that I would not be returning for any more chemotherapy treatments. My belief was firm—I trusted that God had healed me.

Dr. Hacker was already aware of the strength behind my conviction. During our conversation, he spoke gently and compassionately, asking if I would consider undergoing just one more treatment. He suggested that after this session, the three of us—God, Dr. Hacker, and myself—could "shake hands" and agree to move forward together, honoring both my faith and his medical expertise knowing his would not have been his choice decision. I felt sad as if I fell him, but it had taken it told on me. Sadness weighed heavily on me, as though I had let him down. The emotional burden was overwhelming, and I could feel the toll it had taken on my spirit. Each day, the strain became more apparent, and I grappled with the sense of loss and disappointment that lingered within me.

Six-Month Return and Final Surgery Second look laparotomy 6-23-83

SURGEON: Neville Hacker, M.D

IST ASST. SURGEON: Jonathan Berek, M.D

ASST. SURGON: Alan Munoz, M.D

                               Kieth Teraza, M.D

                               Duke Johnson M.S

My follow-up included exploration surgery six months later. They reminded me how important it was not to miss it. I promised to return.

When I arrived back at UCLA, emotion flooded me. The memories of my first day there—the fear, the uncertainty—contrasted with the strength I now carried. Bea told me I would one day ask God for the gift I had been afraid to accept. Now I understand.

A Moment of Honesty

Before the surgery, I felt compelled to share something deeply personal with Dr. Hacker: I revealed that my boyfriend had been married throughout our relationship. Dr. Hacker listened with genuine compassion and encouraged me to choose forgiveness.

This revelation left me questioning why God had allowed such a painful truth to surface during a time when I was already so vulnerable. Yet, with reflection, I came to understand we never had intercourse due to my illness that not everything in life is meant for us to comprehend. I decided to wish him well and move forward, he was there for a reason in a season trusting that God does not hold us accountable for things we do not know. It is what we do when we know.

"Godspeed," I told him.

No Regrets, No 'Why Me,' No Questions, No Replacements

As I reflect on my journey:

- **No regrets**
- **No 'why me'**
- **No questions asked**
- **No replacements**

Everyone who walked this path with me was chosen. Every moment mattered. Every hardship had purpose. And every person at UCLA is etched into my heart forever.

I would not trade any part of this journey. Together, we accomplished something extraordinary. I am honored to have been part of a mission greater than myself.

Chapter 16:
Understanding the Impact of
Family on Personal Growth

Over the years, I have often listened to people express a desire to change their parents or siblings, believing that everything in their lives would be different if only their family members behaved differently. But I have come to realize that changing them would mean living someone else's life, not my own. The truth is that our family shapes us. Altering those relationships would fundamentally change who we are.

Through therapy at a young age, I gained valuable insight into my personal journey. I came to understand that my path would never mirror that of my siblings or friends. Each person's experiences and challenges are unique, and trying to fit in where I did not belong only left me feeling lost and eager to please others. Accepting this allowed me to grow and begin appreciating the distinct course my life was meant to take.

I am grateful for what therapy revealed in me—insights I could not put together on my own. Knowing that you are different is one thing, but truly understanding and accepting those differences is something else entirely. This was a time of important growth for me. As I reflect on this portion of my life, I can see that my journey was not finished. God had many tasks for me—becoming a mother to my father, a mother to my brothers' and sisters' children. The journey continued, and it was the hardest thing I've ever endured.

Reflections on Childhood: Finding Safety Behind the Door

As I look back on my life beginning around age four, I can clearly see who I was and why I struggled to communicate with those around me. Growing up in a home filled with so many older and taller people was overwhelming. Their constant instructions— telling me what to do or not do—made me feel the need to protect myself by keeping my distance.

Bea, my mother, was fearless, and her children were just as boisterous. Arguments and fights broke out regularly, not only among her children but also with other teenagers. The chaos frightened me deeply. When I screamed from behind the door, they told me to stop, not realizing that my cries were rooted in fear. I was terrified they might hurt one another, and I wanted to shield myself from both the sights and sounds of their conflicts.

That door became my refuge—my safe place. It was the only spot where I could retreat unseen and try to process what I was feeling. Even at a young age, I sensed that something about me was different. It wasn't just shyness. I felt fear not only of outsiders, but also of many people in my own home.

Reflections on My Older Self

Looking back on those days, I wish I could tell my younger self—and the older women around me—that what they saw in me was truly a gift. My eyes, which seemed to frighten them, held something special that I didn't recognize until I needed it most. Despite my fear and feelings of being different, there was a strength inside me waiting to be uncovered.

Bea, my mother, fought a good fight so that I might one day understand God's gift. Her anger toward me may have come from sensing that I would eventually ask God for what I once refused to accept. (She knew).

Acknowledgment

Acknowledgment of Divine Guidance: Gratitude for God's Grace

It is with profound gratitude that I acknowledge the essential role of God's grace and mercy in the creation of this book. Without divine guidance and purpose, these pages would never have come to life. This writing journey has been shaped by moments of reflection, correction, and surrender, with the understanding that this book ultimately belongs to its true Author—God.

All glory and praise belong to Him, for it is through faith that healing becomes possible. Without faith, there can be no healing; without healing, this story would remain untold. I am deeply thankful to God for His unwavering presence through every step of this journey.

Tribute to My Mother, Bea

I extend heartfelt thanks to my mother, Bea, for imparting the wisdom and knowledge of God's gift. The journey we traveled together was difficult—a journey that continued "until the wheels rolled off." From the day I was born, you sensed something different in me and did your best to guide me.

In the end, as you predicted, I came to ask God for the gift I once rejected. I now understand the traumas and pain you endured, fighting in the best way you knew how, trying not to lose your children to the streets of Mississippi. Our journey was quite a ride.

Though I did not always understand your choices as I grew into womanhood, I now see that you were trying to protect your daughters from the hardships you faced with unworthy men. I am sorry for the loss of love and respect that left you unwell.

Your Twelve & Se7vn.

Tribute to My Dad: The Final Journey

In those final hours, Dad, I had already packed the car and desperately needed sleep. I had not slept in two days, consumed by a sense of emptiness and searching for answers about what God was revealing to me. Though I didn't understand it, I felt something unknown lingering.

When the call came from the coroner's office, I recognized it as God unveiling His purpose—a reminder that He continually desires to make Himself known. I saw the wave of your hand as you said goodbye. That image remains with me—a still picture marking the completion of your story.

Dad, thank you for being there for Bea. Your presence meant the world to her, especially knowing her husband was by her side in the end. For that, I am deeply grateful.

A Reflection on Grandma Mae, My Father, and Family History

Growing up, Grandma Mae was everything to me—her love and guidance shaped my early life. But as I learned more about our family's history, I discovered a difficult truth. In a moment of anger or frustration, she struck my father in the ear with a shovel. The injury was significant, but he never received medical care for it. This likely contributed to his hearing loss.

Later in life, my father shared how the loud, constant ringing in his ear became unbearable. This persistent noise was one reason he began drinking at a young age. The untreated injury followed him throughout his life, and alcohol became his way of silencing the pain.

Understanding this gave me deeper insight into my father's struggles—and the generational hardships that shaped our family.

Tribute to My Sister, Gloria Montgomery (Missie)

Gloria Montgomery—my beloved sister, Missie—thank you for opening my eyes to a world beyond Mississippi. That visit to Oklahoma with you marked a turning point for me; I realized then that I was destined to see more of the world, and, indeed, I did. My life began to change in ways I could not have imagined.

Joining you and your family in San Bernardino, California was a pivotal moment in my journey. I truly believe that had I not made that choice, I would not be here today. It was more than coincidence—it was part of a greater plan, written from the beginning. God chose this path for me, knowing I had the strength to withstand whatever came my way.

Peace & Love, Gloria Montgomery

Tribute to My Sister-in-Law Eva Curtis

Eva Curtis, my sister-in-law, your unwavering support has meant so much to me, especially as you navigated your own difficult life changes. Despite the challenges you faced, you still cared for me and gave all that you could. For me, that is more than enough, and I want you to know that I have no regrets. I deeply appreciate the journey you walk with me. Your accomplishments shine through, and your perseverance inspires others.

Peace & Love, Eva Curtis

Tribute to Brother-in-Law Retired SMG Air Force

To my brother-in-law, Chester Montgomery —words cannot express the depth of gratitude I feel for all that you gave. You went above and beyond; your support and encouragement were never required, yet you offered them wholeheartedly. Through your guidance, I was able to pursue meaningful opportunities with both the U.S. Air Force and the U.S. Army. You recognized potential in me that I had yet to discover within myself, and your belief fueled my growth and confidence.

As you rest in peace, I honor your legacy of service. You served your country with dedication, and I strive to serve those who have served, finding balance in our shared purpose.

Special Thanks to My Niece Kawanda Curtis Miller

I want to express my deepest gratitude to my niece, Kawanda Miller. Your prayer over me during my illness touched my soul in ways I cannot fully describe. Even at a young age, while still a college student, you possessed an extraordinary gift for prayer— one that cannot be taught or given, but is simply innate. Your heartfelt words and unwavering faith provided me with remarkable strength and reassurance, reminding me through every difficult moment that I was never truly alone.

Special Thanks to My Niece Sheila Curtis Bryant

To my niece, Sheila Bryant: You have always shown wisdom far beyond your years. This rare quality is one of the reasons why your mother, my sister Katie, placed such deep trust in you, especially during those times when Bea needed someone by her side through illness and hardship. Your steady presence and unwavering support brought comfort not only to Bea, but also to our entire family, including my mother and your grandmother. Your quiet strength and compassion made a difference in the lives of those who needed it most, and your role in our family's journey will always be remembered and cherished.

Special Thanks to Paul E Jones,

We are all inherently good people, yet it is important to acknowledge that none of us are perfect. As human beings, we are bound to make mistakes—sometimes good, sometimes bad. What truly matters is how we respond to these experiences: when we know better, we strive to do better, just as the Bible teaches. We must remember that everyone errs, and no one is without fault. As it is written, this wisdom reminds us to approach one another with understanding, compassion, and forgiveness. Made God continue to bless you, my friend.

Enduring Friendship

In life, as we all know, we may encounter many friends, yet only one friend will truly stand the test of time. Some people are not fortunate enough to experience such a lasting connection. I feel blessed to have experienced this kind of friendship. I have never questioned our ability to meet others, always knowing that no matter who might come along, in the end it would be you and I Portia Maria Stringer. My bestie, roll until the wheel ran off. RIP.

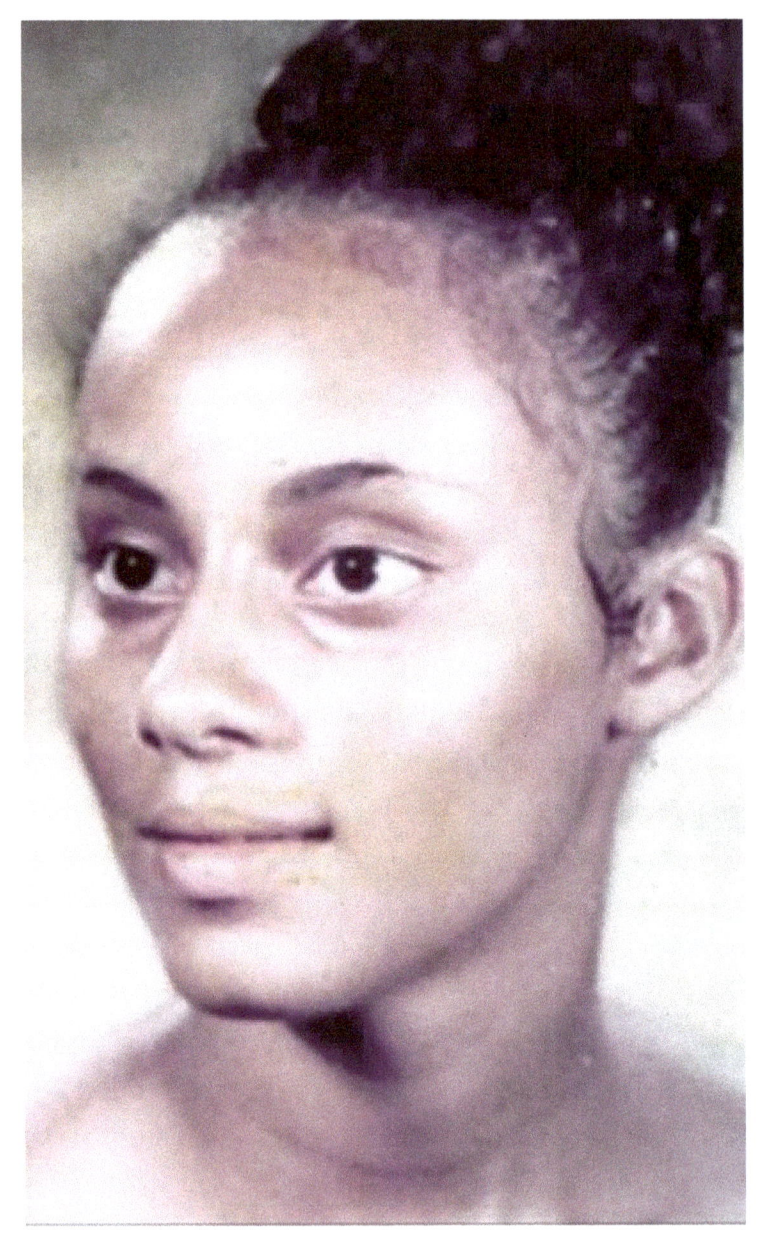

Dr. Luke Hsiao: The Surgeon

Dr. Luke Hsiao: A Beacon of Hope During My Struggles

During one of the most vulnerable periods of my life, I was blessed to encounter Dr. Luke Hsiao. His compassion and unwavering determination left an indelible mark on me, shaping my journey in ways I will never forget.

Dr. Hsiao's Unwavering Commitment and Compassion

A Surgeon's Dedication Beyond Expertise

When a surgeon encounters a challenge that surpasses their own expertise, their true dedication to patient care is revealed. Rather than accepting defeat, a surgeon seeks out more qualified colleagues to ensure the best possible outcome. I am profoundly grateful that God blessed Dr. Hsiao with both the vision and humility to reach out for additional help on my behalf. His commitment to my well-being demonstrated exceptional care and perseverance. Dr. Hsiao never gave up on me, and for that, I am deeply and honorably grateful. Simply put, Dr. Hsiao, you are the best.

Searching the World for Hope

Dr. Hsiao devoted himself wholeheartedly to my care, tirelessly searching worldwide for someone who had survived at least one year with the rare cancer I faced. The countless hours he spent seeking hope for me showed a level of dedication and compassion that was truly extraordinary.

The Moment of Hope

I am certain that without Dr. Hsiao's diligent efforts, I would not be here today. When he finally gathered my family together, he entered the room with a smile that lit up the entire space. I still remember his uplifting words: "Little Girl, there is hope. I found someone. They're waiting for you. Please take it."

A Source of Strength

His unwavering support became my foundation of strength. As a young Black girl from Mississippi, receiving this depth of care and belief meant everything to me. In times when I felt alone and isolated, Dr. Hsiao's kindness served as a powerful reminder that I was never truly by myself.

To Dr. Hsiao—you will always be my angel.

God bless you, my angel.

Your Little Girl.

Professor Neville Hacker

2 October1982, I arrived at UCLA Medical Center,

ADIMISSION DIAGNOSIS: Endodermal sinus tumor, Stage III. (Germ Cell Tumor)

Our journey began with a simple knock at the door, followed by a unique voice asking, "Can we come in?" I said yes, and a group of doctors in white coats entered my room. That moment will stay with me forever. With a warm smile and a gentle greeting, Dr. Neville Hacker introduced himself. There were so many faces and names, but his stood out above all.

Finding Family in Unexpected Places

He recognized my vulnerability immediately, as tears welled up in my eyes. Understanding that I was alone, without my mother or father, Dr. Hacker and his team became the family I needed most. It felt as if only God could have provided such support for me during one of the most emotional periods of my life, at just 23 years old.

In those moments of deep loneliness and uncertainty, Dr. Hacker's compassion was unwavering. The absence of my parents left a void, but the kindness and presence of the medical team helped fill that emptiness. Their support was not just professional—it was profoundly personal, providing comfort and reassurance when I needed it most. Surrounded by caring individuals who treated me with empathy and respect, I found the strength to face the challenges ahead. This sense of family, forged in a hospital room, became a source of hope and resilience during a time when I felt most vulnerable.

Empathy Beyond Diagnosis

Dr. Hacker's empathy reached beyond the boundaries of the cancer diagnosis; he saw the pain in my heart and was genuinely concerned about my overall well-being. Receiving a serious medical diagnosis is emotionally overwhelming, bringing waves of fear, sadness, and uncertainty about the future. The concern for loved ones, combined with the reality of illness, creates a complex emotional experience. In these moments, the support and compassion of both family and medical professionals are essential, helping to provide strength and reassurance when it is needed most.

During my time at the hospital, you and your medical team remained by my bedside, gently talking with me and offering comfort. While Dr. Hacker and other members of the team discussed my case nearby, I never felt alone; instead, I felt surrounded by genuine care and concern. Soon, everyone gathered around me, making it clear that I now had the support of a family. Their presence and compassion gave me the strength I needed to face the challenges ahead.

Our conversations were reassuring, leaving no questions unanswered and instilling confidence in me. Throughout my treatment, your unwavering belief in my ability to overcome obstacles never wavered, and my faith remained strong. I truly felt that God had a hand in my healing, guiding me through each step of the journey.

Reflecting on these moments, I realize that if our paths had not crossed, this story would never have been written. I have never forgotten you over the years Professor Hacker and the team you put together. Many distinguished gastrointestinal and gynecological specialists have overseen my health since then, and all have been fascinated by the guidance and support I received during that time. There was even a time when what you did was described as putting together an atlas—now, they call it a navigation system. Because of you, I have met incredible people who have all wanted to witness your remarkable work and talents. Professor Hacker, not surprised of your accomplishments" suggests that the individual always possessed a high level of intelligence, diligence, or ambition, making their significant achievements seem like a natural and expected progression of their career. My Angel

Thank You for an amazing ride. May heaven and earth continue to bless you and your family!!

Gratitude for Prayers and Support

I am deeply grateful for all the prayers, love, and support I received throughout my journey. Each call and message I received meant so much to me, serving as a reminder that I was surrounded by a caring community. Knowing that you were praying for me brought immense comfort during the most difficult times. The power of prayer truly lifted my spirit and helped me keep faith as I faced my illness.

The Girl Behind the Door: A Memoir of Family, Faith, and Resilience

This memoir traces the arc of my life from the bustling heart of Madea's home in Clarksdale, Mississippi, through trials, tragedies, and triumphs, to healing and self-discovery in California. It is a story of family, faith, and the search for identity amidst chaos. The chapters are drawn from vivid memories, moments of quiet reflection, and the enduring hope that even in the darkest places, a gift awaits. I invite you to walk with me through these pivotal years and witness the resilience that grows from the roots of love and pain.

Clarksdale, Mississippi was a tapestry of kinship, stitched together by the hands of Madea—the family matriarch who infused her home with warmth, tradition, and the gentle authority that shaped generations. Her days began early, filled with routines of kneading dough, folding laundry, and guiding her grandchildren with a soft, unwavering voice. Holiday celebrations and daily visits from children and grandchildren made her house the center of gravity, a sanctuary where laughter mingled with tears and stories stitched the fragments of memory into the fabric of family strength.

The loss of Madea—and Grandaddy before her—left a void that grief could not fill. Yet, the foundation of kindness and love they built endured, guiding us through sorrow and into gratitude for the memories they left behind. Their legacy became a bedrock of belonging, anchoring us through seasons of change.

Chapter 1: The Girl Behind the Door

Before I turned four, every morning began with a visit to Madea's house. My mother, Bea, orchestrated the day, her call for Shirley Jean signaling the start. I was the "baby chick," quiet and timid, often found in my favorite spot behind the door—seeking comfort in solitude while Shirley Jean helped me manage the ache in my knees and the confusion of home. It was here, in the hush of shadows, that I learned the meaning of safety and the beginnings of withdrawal from chaos.

Chapter 2: Twists & Secrets

Family rituals unfolded in the rhythms of weekend visits, code word games, and the rituals of kindness that lingered after Madea's passing. Secrets were woven through these traditions—quiet gestures, hidden fears, and the unspoken rules of belonging. I navigated the tensions between siblings, the enigmatic words of town ladies, and the mysteries of "the gift" that set me apart, even as friendship began to blossom outside my door.

Chapter 3: Contest of Endurance & Holiday Triumph

Community events became a stage for family resilience: Thanksgiving gatherings, the anticipation of the Christmas truck contest, and the parade that united us in pride and celebration. The contest tested our endurance and willpower, bringing excitement and hope—especially as Dad's victory became a symbol of triumph after hardship. Through holidays and contests, we found unity amidst loss and the quiet strength to carry forward.

Chapter 4: Sundays Faith & Family

Sundays in our home began with Bea's voice singing "Amazing Grace," a routine of preparation for church, and the shared responsibilities that brought order to chaos. Faith and scripture shaped our evenings, as friendly competitions over biblical passages fostered camaraderie and deeper understanding. Yet, behind the door, I continued to seek solace, listening and longing for the peace that came only on Sundays.

Chapter 5: The Womb

Trauma found me in the form of family conflict and a violent incident that left scars both physical and emotional. The pain and confusion from my brother's actions, the silence that followed, and the struggle to find safety behind the door defined my early healing. Support came from Shirley Jean and Dr. Burnham, whose concern for my well-being offered a glimmer of understanding and the first steps toward recovery.

Chapter 6: Finding My Way in First Grade

School was a new world—filled with challenges, bullying, and the fear of exposure. Tears, spankings, and repeated returns to class marked my struggle for acceptance. Yet, friendship became a lifeline, and counseling offered a path toward healing. The journey from fear to confidence was slow, but each small victory—birthday parties, homework, and the reassurance of my friends—began to shape a sense of belonging and hope.

Chapter 7: Family Dynamics, Loss, and Growth

Loss and adaptation were constants in our family. Siblings moved away, relationships shifted, and the absence of Grandma Mae echoed through our routines. Bea's rules clashed with Dad's habits, and the dynamics of discipline, blame, and autonomy created tension and isolation. Through therapy and reflection, I began to understand my own boundaries and the need for acceptance amidst the chaos.

Chapter 8: Eyes of the Unknown

Community perceptions colored my self-discovery. The town's ladies warned Bea about my eyes, speaking in hushed tones about "the gift" I carried. Their fear and avoidance left me questioning my identity, searching for meaning in the mysteries that set me apart. Bea's advice to focus on God and gratitude offered comfort, but the longing for understanding remained.

Chapter 9: Tragedy & Tragic

Tragedy struck when a fire claimed the life of my niece and shattered the sense of security we once knew. Loss scattered our family, forcing separation and adaptation. Grief was compounded by Bea's explanations of heaven, the inevitability of death, and the challenge of coping with absence. Through faith and the support of family, we learned to gather strength and move forward.

Chapter 10: Discovering Who I Am

Adolescence brought independence, therapy, and the struggle to assert my voice amid family criticism and discipline. Encounters with authority, conflict with siblings, and the journey through counseling revealed a deeper understanding of my own resilience and the necessity of leaving Mississippi to find my place in the world. Outgrowing the limitations of home, I embraced my difference as strength.

Chapter 11: The Path to Independence

Coming of age meant longing for freedom, new experiences, and the chance to leave home. Oklahoma and Chicago offered glimpses of independence, the challenges of adulthood, and the bittersweet lessons of growing up—no longer relying on family, but learning to stand on my own. Mistakes, embarrassment, and survival shaped the journey, leading to self-sufficiency and pride.

Chapter 12: Bea's Life Before and After Cancer

Bea's journey as a young mother was marked by sacrifice, reliance on Madea and Grandaddy, and the cycle of support that defined our family. Her strength was tested by cancer, and the family rallied around her during illness and recovery. The experience of caring for Bea, reflecting on her wisdom, and understanding the depth of her struggles deepened my appreciation for the legacy she left behind.

Chapter 13: Warning Before the Storm

Relocation to California brought new opportunities, friendships, and the challenge of self-discovery. Technical school, work, and social circles became the backdrop for personal growth and the pursuit of healing after Bea's passing. The resilience forged in family adversity carried me forward into new environments and the start of a career.

Chapter 14: Chosen Cancer

Diagnosis with terminal cancer was a turning point—marked by fear, confusion, and the search for meaning. The journey through surgery, faith, and the support of Dr. Hsiao and Dr. Hacker revealed the power of hope, prayer, and divine intervention. The battle with chemotherapy, the decision to trust in healing, and the lessons learned in survival became a testament to resilience and faith.

Chapter 15: Welcome to UCLA

The medical journey at UCLA was a story of healing and support—a family of doctors, nurses, and caregivers who carried me through the darkest hours. Recovery was marked by milestones, setbacks, and the importance of mental health and therapy. The compassion of Dr. Hacker and the encouragement of the team restored my sense of hope, leading to lasting healing and gratitude.

Chapter 16: Understanding the Impact of Family on Personal Growth

6honor my differences, grow beyond the need to please others, and recognize the unique path I was meant to travel. Looking back, I see the gift that fear, pain, and resilience have given me—an understanding that my story is my own, and that healing is possible.

Epilogue: Lessons Learned, Legacy, and Hope

As I close this chapter, I am grateful for the journey that has brought me here—the lessons learned in sorrow and joy, the legacy of faith and resilience, and the hope that guides me forward. This memoir is a testament to the enduring power of family, the gift of healing, and the possibility of transformation. May every reader find comfort, strength, and inspiration in these pages—and may you discover your own gift, waiting quietly behind the door.

Acknowledgments and Tributes

Special thanks to my mother Bea, my father, sisters, brothers, nieces, nephews, and all the family members whose stories are woven through this book. To the medical teams who became family in my time of need—your compassion and care will never be forgotten. To friends and loved ones who prayed, supported, and believed in me, this story is yours as much as mine.

References (if applicable)

This memoir is based on personal experiences, family stories, and recollections. Medical details are drawn from patient records, personal conversations, and the support of UCLA Medical Center staff.

All chapter titles, headings, and transitions have been clarified for narrative flow and thematic consistency. The author's voice is preserved, with transitions and structural organization enhanced for clarity and coherence. The manuscript is formatted according to standard submission guidelines for memoirs, with double-spaced text, clear chapter divisions, and consistent narrative style.

Your Twelve & Se7vn

The journey through life has often been marked by significant numbers Twelve and Seven—that carry deep meaning and personal significance. These numbers represent milestones, challenges, and the unique path that has shaped my experiences and understanding of myself. Each phase, whether it was the number Twelve or Se7vn the trials I faced contributed to the person I am today. They are reminders of the moments that defined my growth, resilience, and the lessons learned along the way.

The '12' basket fish, of left over fish, refers to the miracle of feeding the 5,000.12 baskets left over as described in the Gospels of Matthew, Mark and John. interpreted as symbolizing the 12 disciples or tribes of Israel.

Jerusalem as having 12 gates mentioned in the Old Testament each gate, with three on each side (north, south, east, and west) The twelve tribes of Israel

1. Valley Gate
2. Gate of the Fountain

3. Sheep Gate
4. Fish Hates
5. Old Gates
6. Dung Gate
7. Water Gate
8. Horse Gate
9. East Gate
10. Gate of Miphkad
11. The Gate of Ephraim
12. Prison Gate

The Number 7 in the Bible signifies Completion, Perfection, and Devine Fullness

The number 12 and 7 Meaning Completion

I'm the baby of 12 with my mother and the baby 7 with my father and mother.

Acknowledgment and Reflection on Service

I would like to express my deepest gratitude to the thousands of Military Officers in the US Army Medical Corps. Thank you for your dedicated service; it was truly an honor and a pleasure to serve alongside you all.

At times, I have reflected on my experiences and the impact I may have had, but I know it was never solely my doing. I serve a God who brings blessings and makes things possible. It is through this faith that I recognize the true source of every success and every moment of grace.

Each of you has touched my soul in profound ways. The journey we shared was not just mine, but one guided by God—a journey that encompassed everyone who came through the Basic Officer Leadership Course (BOLC). Your presence and service were part of a greater purpose, and I am deeply grateful for the opportunity to have been part of it.

Preserving Gratitude for the Future

My profound gratitude will be preserved in Volume II. This acknowledgment serves as a testament to the deep appreciation I hold for every individual who has been part of this remarkable journey. By documenting these reflections and expressions of thanks. I aim to ensure that the impact and significance of our shared experiences are never forgotten. This record will stand as a lasting tribute to the dedication, service, and faith that defined our time together.

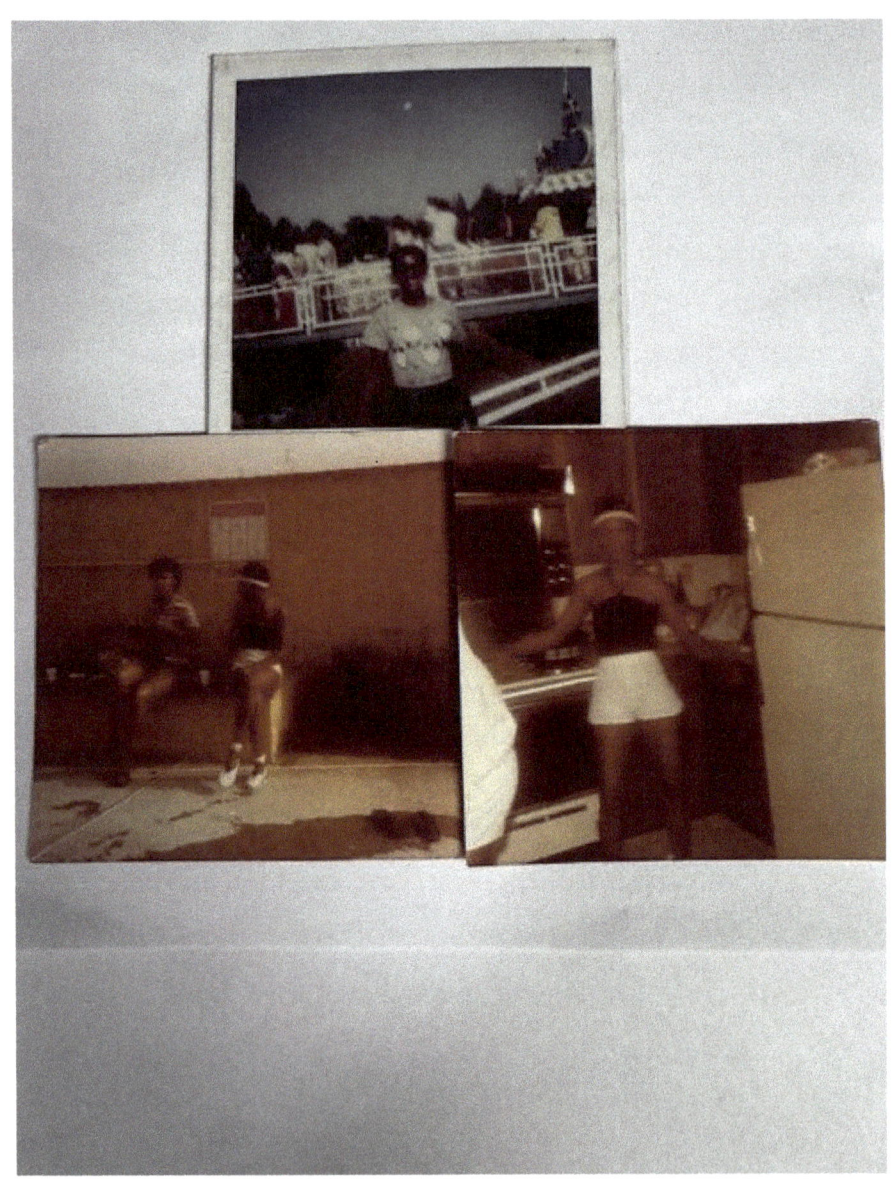

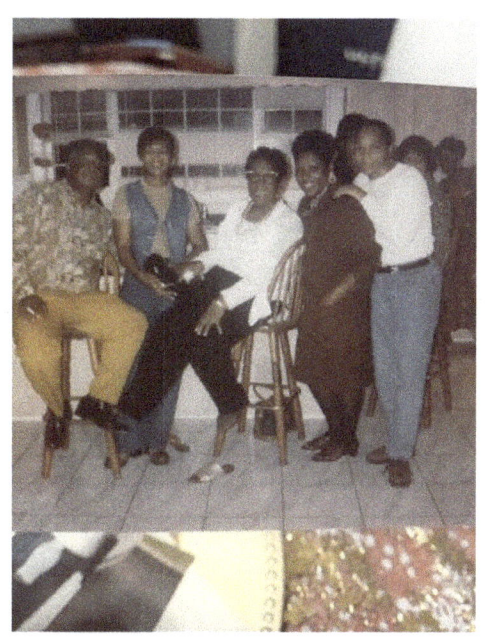

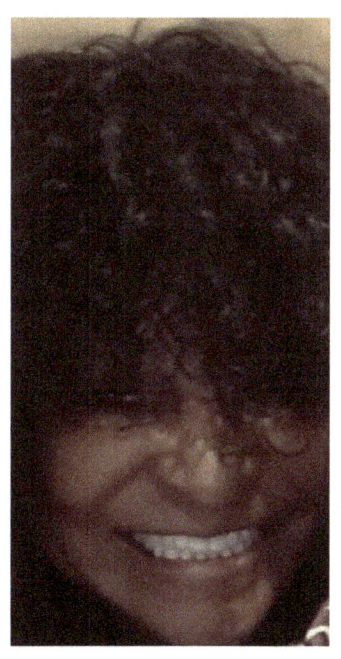

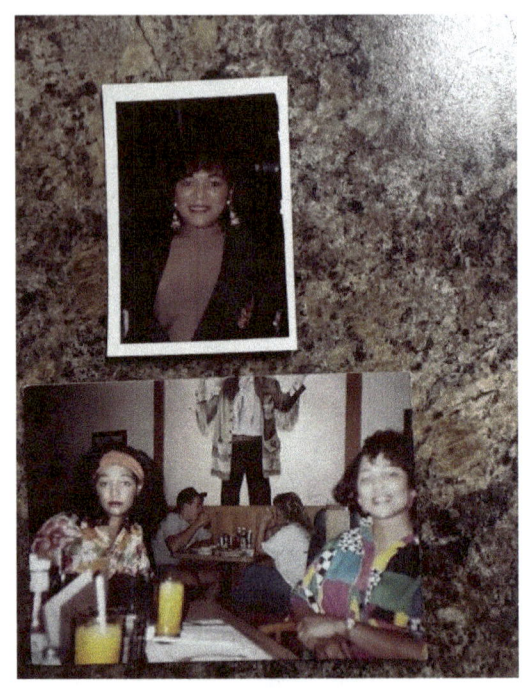

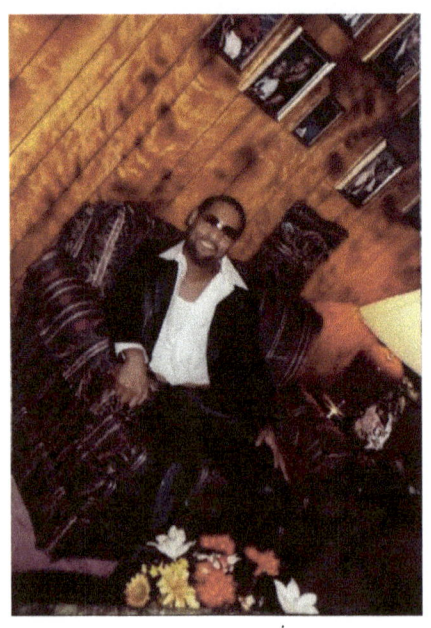

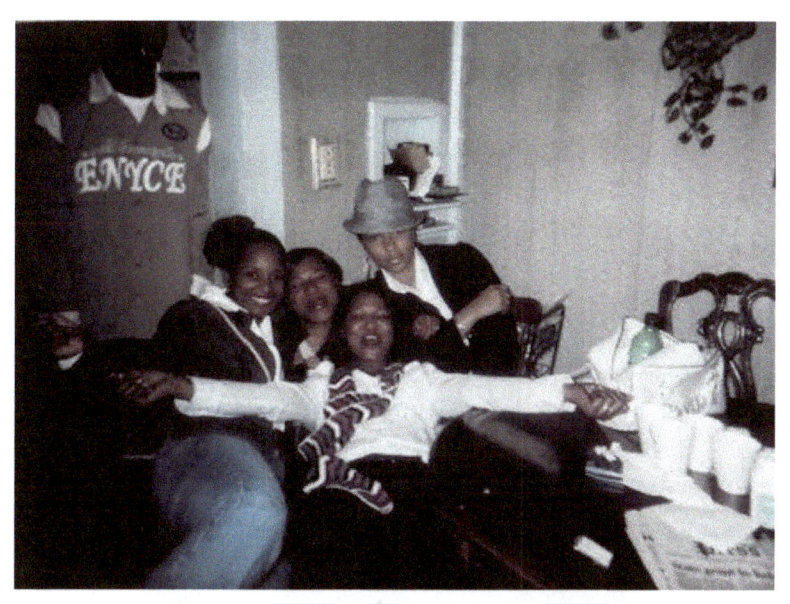

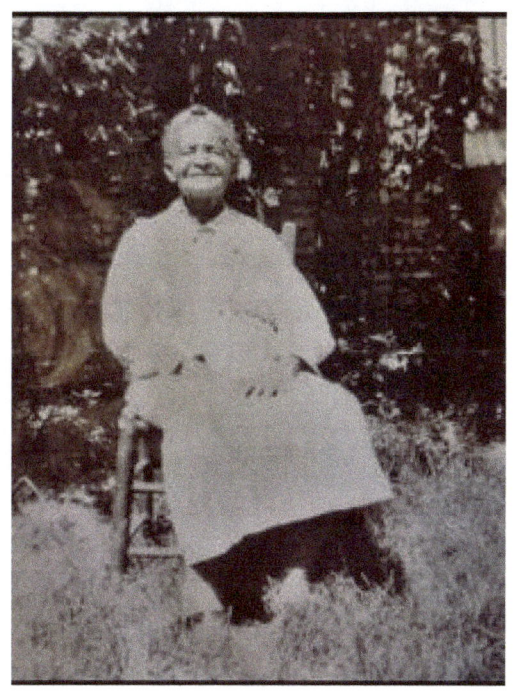

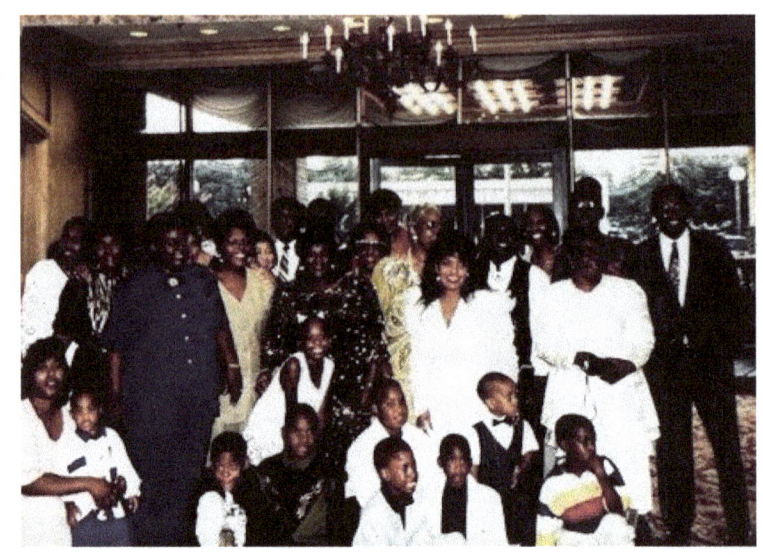

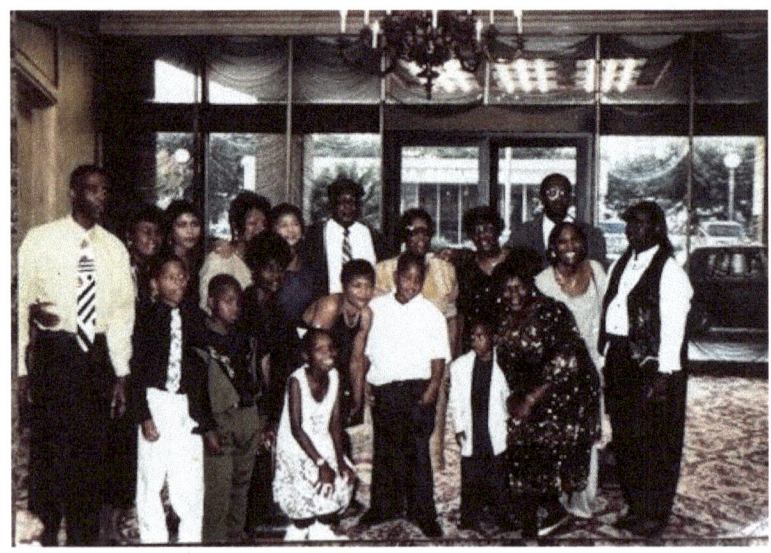

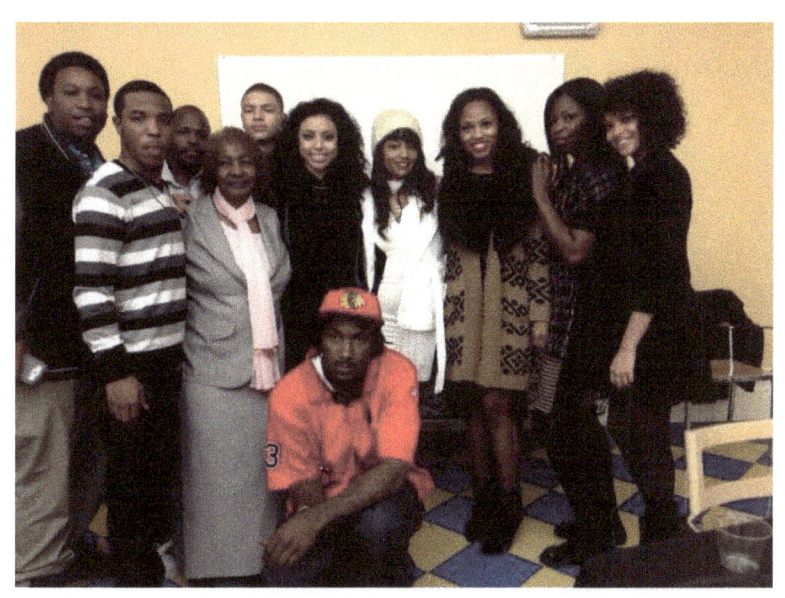

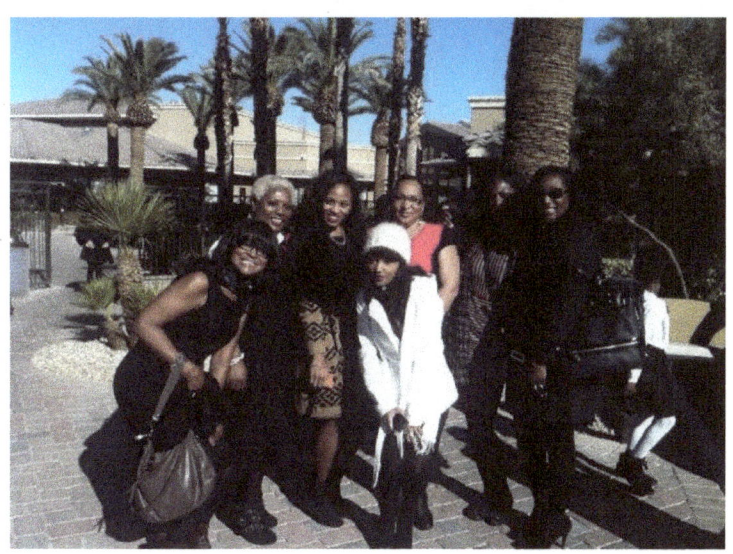

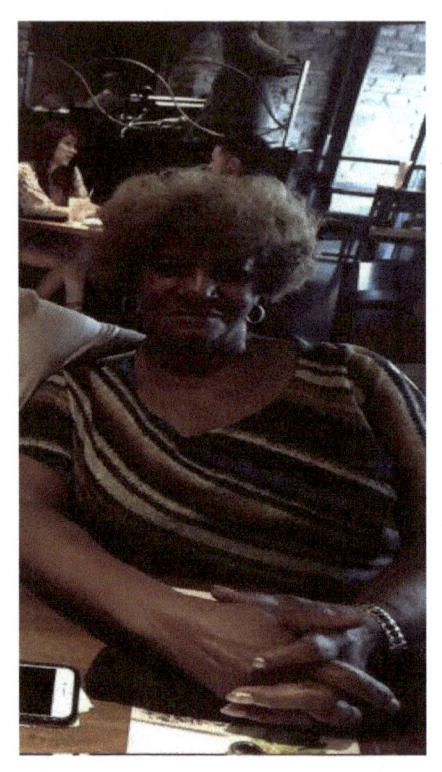

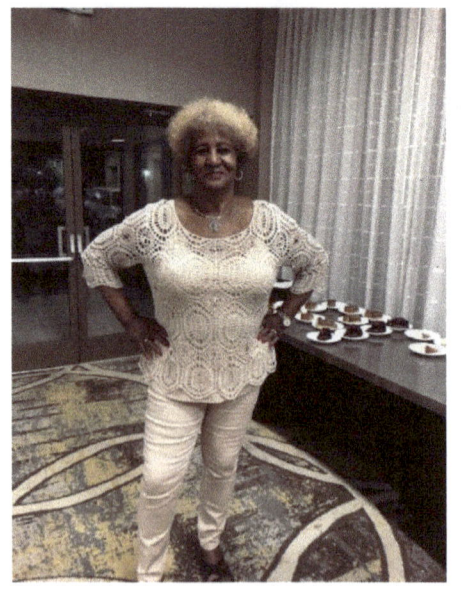

224

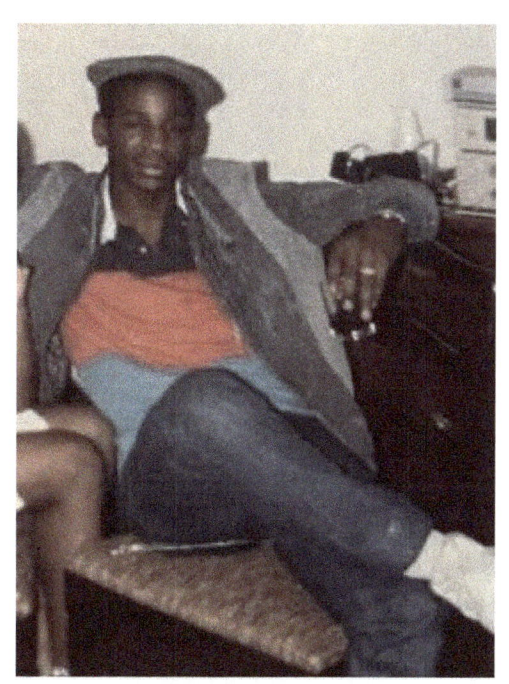

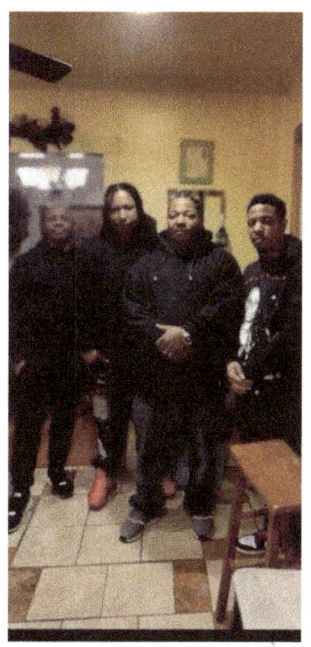

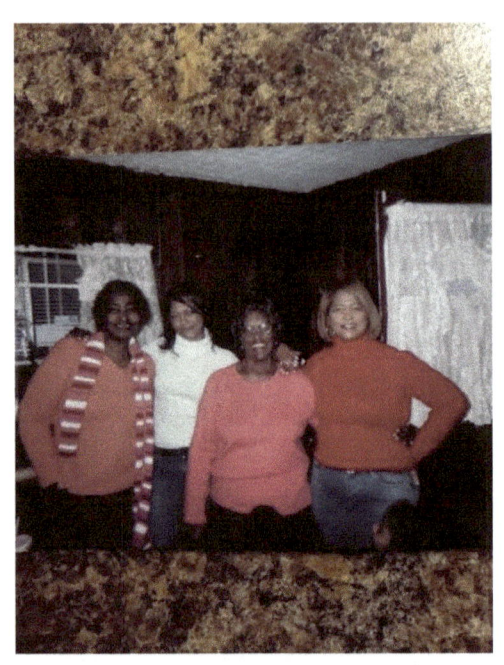

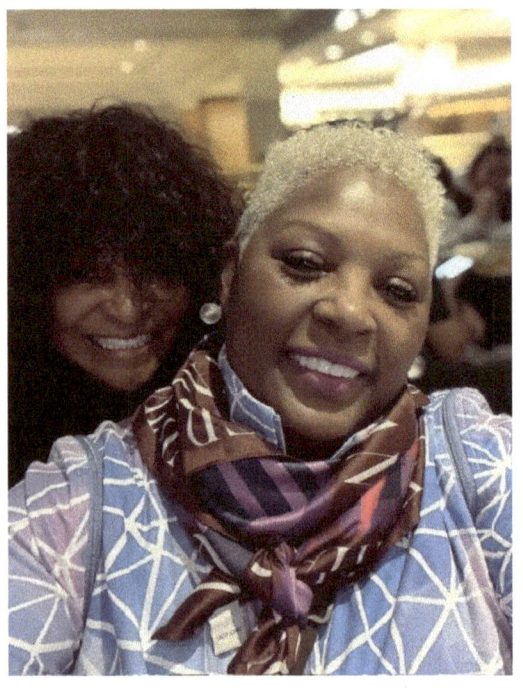

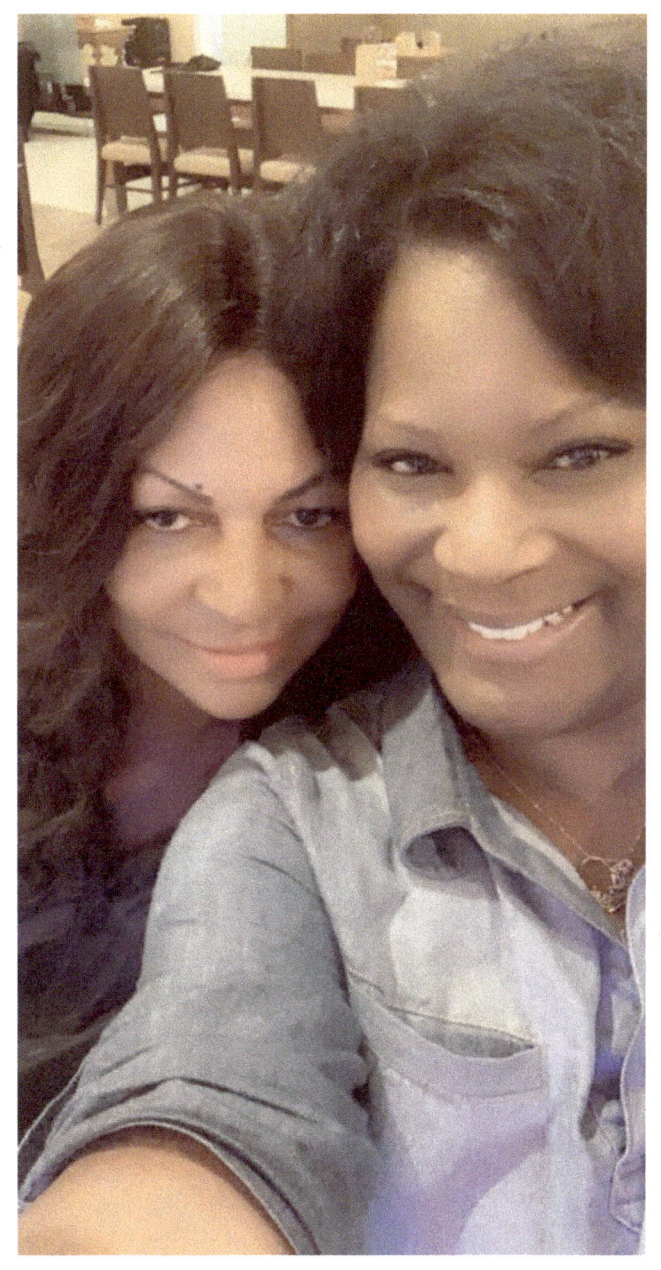

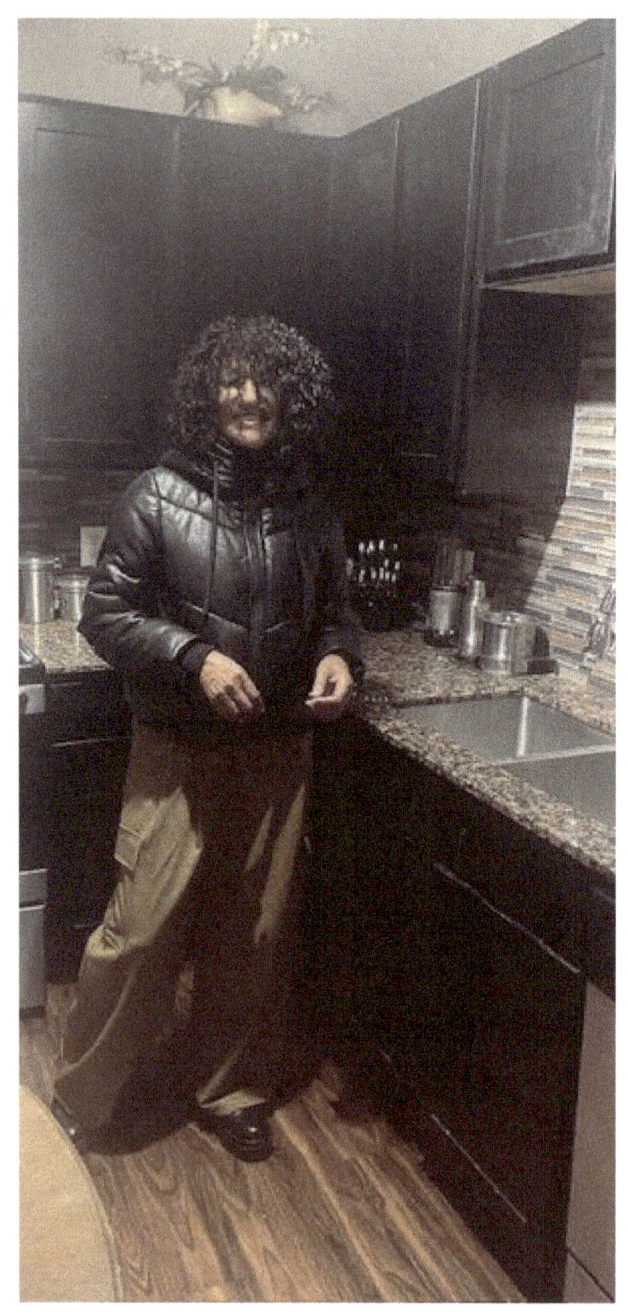

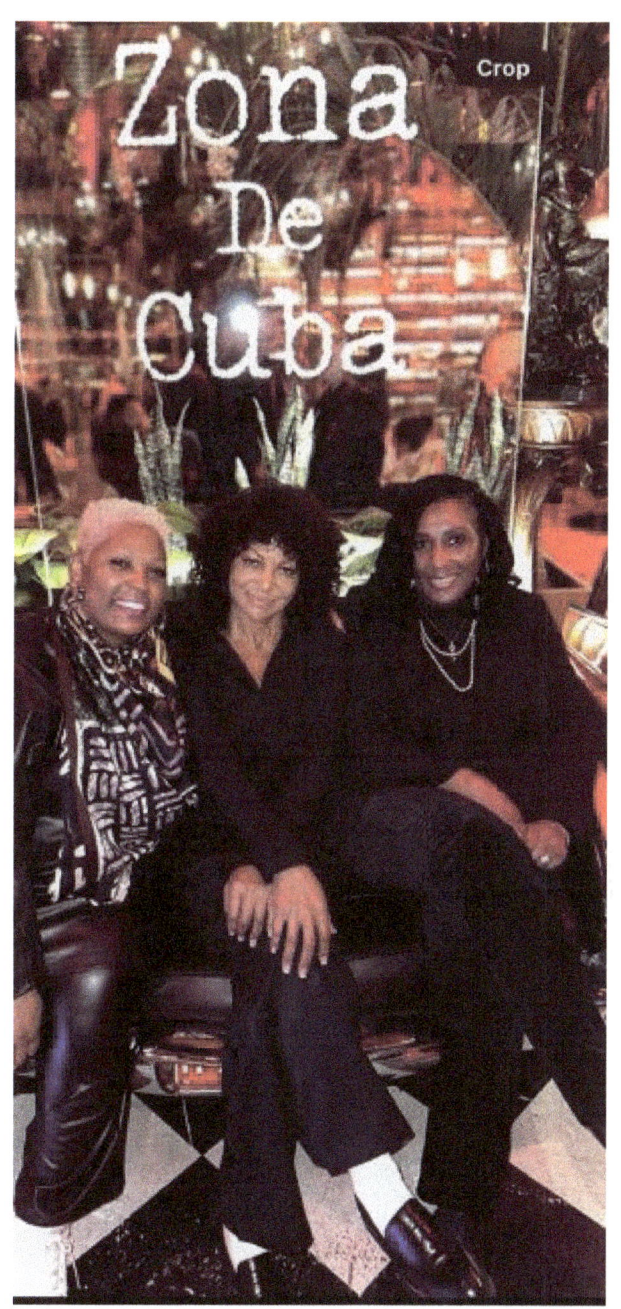

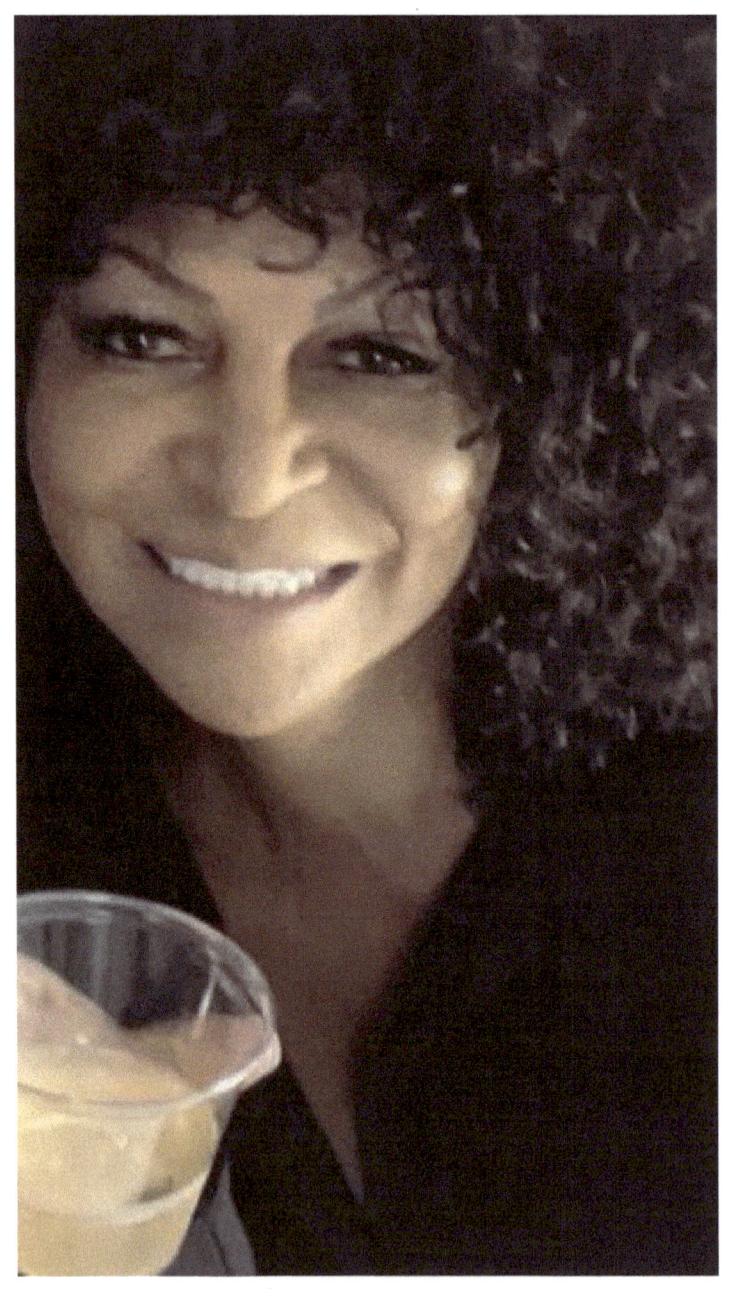

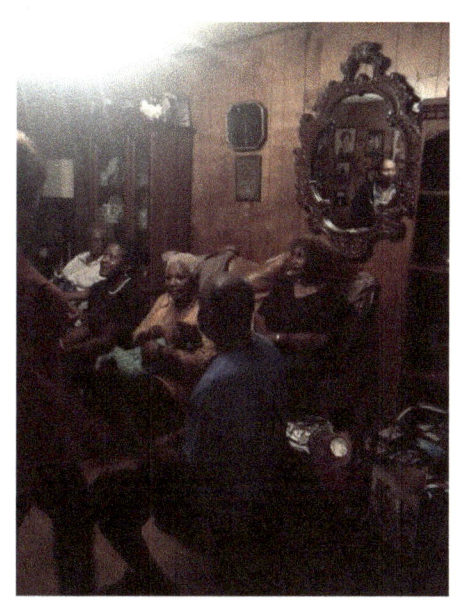

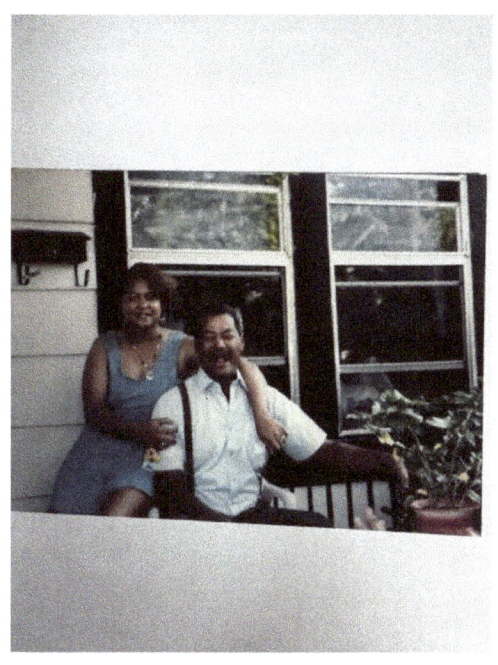

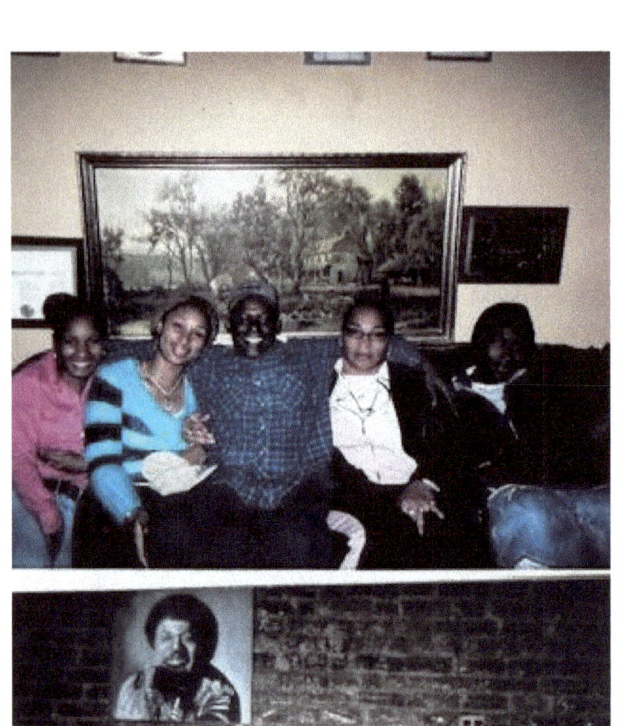

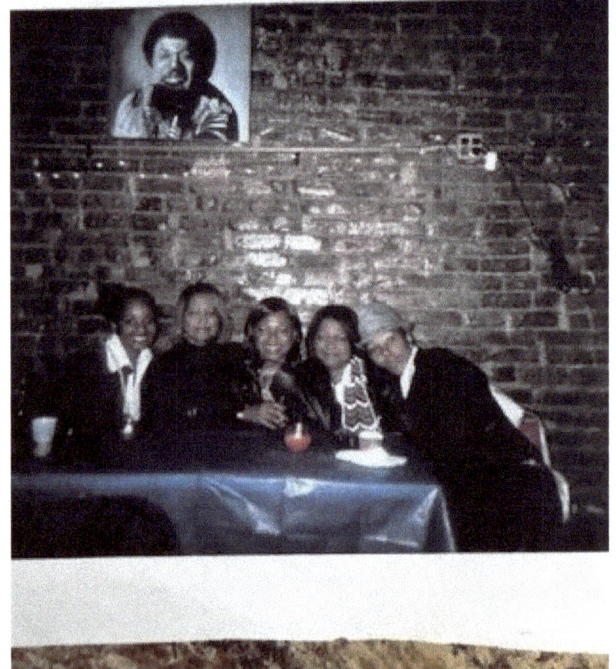

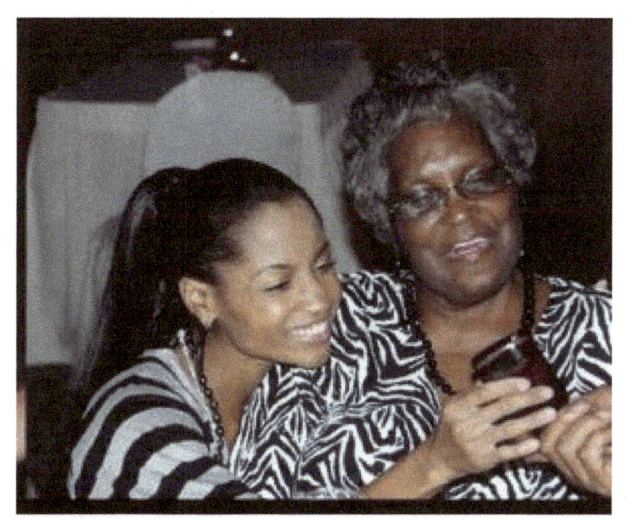

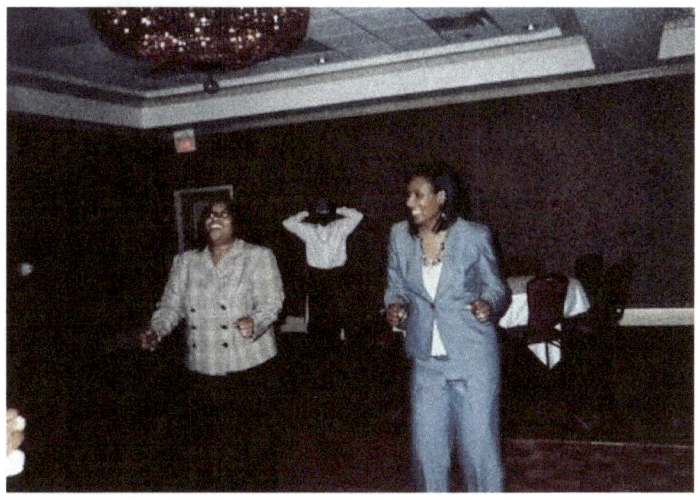

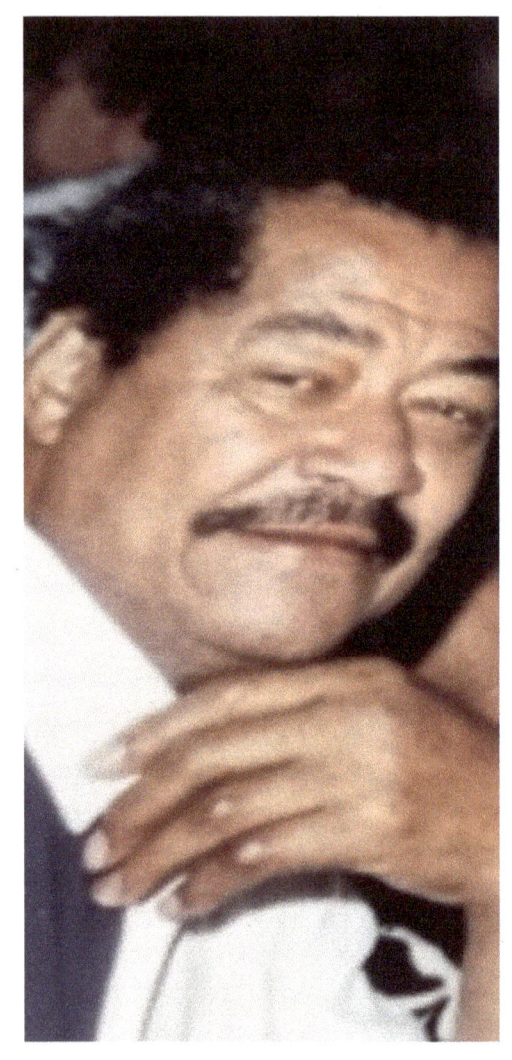

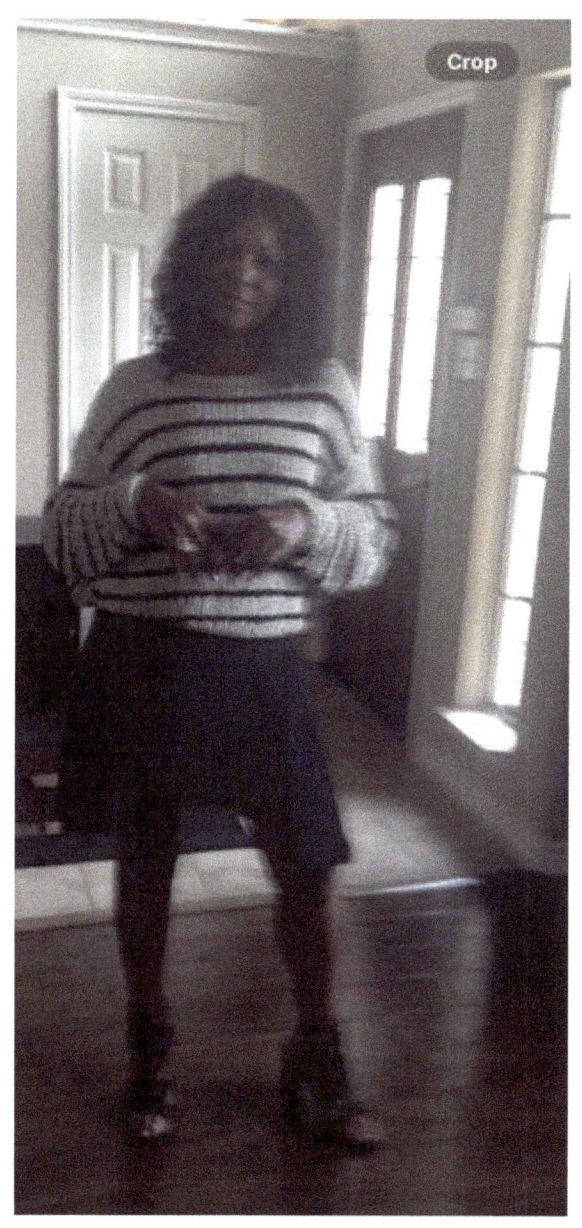

235